Save Your BRAIN

Dr. Michael Colgan

Science Books
Vancouver, BC
2007

Colgan Institute
Ph. 250-537-2069
askdrc@colganinstitute.com
www.colganinstitute.com

Save Your Brain
Science Books/January 2007

This book is not intended for the treatment of disease, nor as a substitute for medical treatment, nor as an alternative to medical advice. It is a review of scientific evidence presented for information purposes, to increase public knowledge of developments in the field of brain chemistry. Although the information contained in this book was prepared from sources that are believed to be accurate and reliable, the publisher strongly advises readers to seek the advice of their personal health care professional(s) before proceeding with any changes in any health care program.

PRE PUBLICATION EDITION

Colgan, Michael, 1939–
    Save Your Brain
Includes bibliographical references and index
ISBN 0-9781794-1-2

BISAC Codes: 0CC 011 000 Healing General;   HEA 039 110
Nevous System;   HEA 017 000 Nutrition   I. Title

Printed in Canada.

Science Books
Vancouver, BC
www.colganinstitute.com

10   9   8   7   6   5   4   3   2   1

To Lesley,
my life partner,
my everything.

Forewords

Sitting quietly between our ears, you and I have our most precious possession — The Brain. Because it doesn't jump up and down and make a noise, we assume that it isn't doing anything very much and so ignore it. Yet, it is the most active organ in the body. Its requirements for fuel and oxygen are prodigious, as is its output. Cutting off its blood supply at normal body temperature for more than five minutes results in brain death, whereas other cells in the body can survive such deprivation many times longer and return to full function when the circulation is restored.

The brain is totally dependent on the body for its essential supplies. If you want to keep your marbles throughout your life (and who doesn't), this book is for you. It incorporates new information on nutrition, a new slant on other works by Dr. Colgan. In addition it emphasizes the need for using one's mental facilities: just as muscle will atrophy when not used, and nourished well, so will brain function fail if not used and nourished adequately and regularly.

Excellent as his other books are, I consider this to be the most important of all Dr. Colgan's writings. Get the book, and don't just sit on it; the seat of learning tends to be a little higher.

Andrew Strigner, MD, Consultant Physician, Harley Street, London, UK

I've known Michael Colgan for many years, and I'm a deep admirer of his approach to living a healthy, nutritionally sound lifestyle. His newest book, *Save your brain*, is a fascinating, yet practical look at how we can improve our single most vital organ – the brain. This book is a must for those who want to improve their intelligence, memory, and their physical function in every aspect of their lives!

Paul Meyer, Founder of Success Motivation International, Inc., and more than 40 other companies and New York Times best-selling author

Dr. Colgan once again presents cutting edge research in a way that is so easy to understand and entertaining to read. His research is meticulous, and right up to date. His work is always eye-opening - he is without a doubt one of the world's leading writers in the fields of nutrition and health.

Phillip Mills, President of Les Mills International Ltd. – world leaders in group fitness; Creator of BODYPUMP™, the world's most popular branded fitness class

In *Save Your Brain* Michael teaches with explicit candor and uncommon clarity not only how to save our brain, but more importantly, why we must. There is no worse disease as Michael states, than to outlive our intelligence. The Brain Program is exactly that; a powerful nutrition strategy that beckons to all inclined by reason and intellect to protect the most important real estate of all; that mysterious grey mass hiding behind the eyes.

Cory Holly, DN, Founder and President of the Cory Holly Institute - Sports Nutrition Education Center

Being in the golf industry for 30 years, I notice the mental decline of my aging members. In addition to general forgetfulness and lack of concentration on the course, Alzheimer's, Parkinson's, Huntington's and other forms of brain degeneration appear commonplace in every club. Memories decline, balance worsens, and forgotten phones numbers and tee times become the norm. After following Dr. Colgan's advice and brain-saving strategies for years, I find myself to be the exception. The results of his tactics are very similar to improving your golf game: start early, continue practicing, and enjoy your results.

Kevin S. Paluch, COO & PGA Professional – Geneva National Golf Club

During the 10 years that I have been practicing anti-aging medicine, Dr. Colgan has been an invaluable resource for my own personal education and as a resource for my patients. During the time I have known Dr. Colgan personally, I have been a fervent follower of his writings, and his long-awaited book on protecting the health of the human brain is a revelation, ahead of its time, and should spark a revolution in the way we approach aging

Charles Myers, MD, Chi3 Wellness Centre

Acknowledgements

As a young researcher in the 1970s, I had the advantage of working with the great Canadian physician Hans Selye, who discovered the relationship between what we now call "stress" and ancient structures in the mid-brain. Since that time many fine researchers, too many to name, have advanced our knowledge of brain function at the Colgan Institute. I will let my thanks to my original mentor stand as thanks to all, in this our first book for the public on the human brain.

I have had tremendous help. My executive Brenda Kennedy worked many extra hours to enable us to get the labor done. Megan Colgan worked tirelessly to perform computer wonders on the manuscript, and drawings. And my dearest partner Lesley held us all together through the heavy bits.

My thanks go most of all to the more than 1500 people who have endured endless testing on successive models of our brain programs over the last two decades, testing that gives me the confidence to put this information before you. These folk are pioneers of the human race, the first with sufficient scientific knowledge to attempt to extend the life of the most important possession you will ever have, that three pounds of living matter between your ears.

Also by Dr. Michael Colgan

Your Personal Vitamin Profile (1982)
Optimum Sports Nutrition (1993)
The New Nutrition (1994)
Hormonal Health (1996)
Beat Arthritis (2000)
Protect Your Prostate (2000)
The New Power Program (2001)
Sports Nutrition Guide (2002)
You Can Prevent Cancer (2007)
Nutrition for Chapions (2007)

Introduction

The origins of this book go back to studies that the Colgan Institute presented at Oxford University in the early '80s. In conjunction with other groups, we gave nutritional supplements to children with diverse types of learning difficulties. Even with the crude information available at that time, results showed significant increases in intelligence and learning.

Our 2006 model of the Brain Program stems from the spectacular advances in understanding of the chemistry of the human brain that have been quietly occurring since the turn oif the millennium in research laboratories worldwide. Especially in the last three years, what is now called the "excitotoxic model of brain dysfunction," represents a leap forward in medicine at least as important as the discovery of antibiotics, and with even greater potential to protect us from disease.

I wish I could claim we worked it all out at the Colgan Institute, but that is not so. For the past quarter century, we have drawn heavily on the findings of medical scientists worldwide to piece together the knowledge underlying this book. We feel it has now reached a stage of development sufficient to present to the public as a scientific strategy to improve intelligence, memory and learning ability, and to protect the brain from neurodegenerative disease.

The major discovery from recent research is that the stresses of modern life damage the brains of almost all apparently healthy people. This damage starts to show at about age 35 as measurable declines in cognition. Inevitable progression of this damage over decades, eventually emerges as neurodegenerative disease, especially Alzheimer's and Parkinson's with progressive losses of intelligence and memory, skilled movement, balance, and organ function, until death relieves the suffering. Not a pretty picture, but one we should act upon quickly, while there is still time enough left in our lives to prevent it.

In the US alone, Alzheimer's, the most common manifestation of brain damage, afflicts nearly five million diagnosed people. Another estimated four million cases remain undiagnosed. Parkinson's, the second most common brain disease, afflicts over one million diagnosed people. Many, many others have similar brain damage, including the mostly undiagnosed damage that occurs in young athletes who fail to fully recover from the overtraining syndrome.

The US Centers for Disease Control in Atlanta, report that half of all Americans living today will spend their latter years in nursing homes, unable to care for themselves. The predominant cause of this incapacity is not a decline in muscle or organ function, but a decline of the mind. Current health policies cannot protect you from this fate. If you want to keep your brain, you have to learn to protect yourself.

We know now that if death from another cause does not intervene, the excitotoxic brain damage of usual aging, finally manifests as Alzheimer's, Parkinson's, Lou Gerhig's disease or other form of neurodegeneration. The particular disease that predominates, depends to a small extent on the genetic inheritance of the person, which makes some cell complexes in the brain more vulnerable than others. Nevertheless, the latest research shows clearly, that brain disease depends most on the particular toxins and traumas and nutritional deficits, to which the individual's brain is exposed during life.

The most exciting discovery is: although symptoms may differ, all common brain diseases share many of the same underlying causes. Therefore all can be inhibited, or even prevented by the same strategies. Save Your Brain combines the best and safest of these strategies, into one powerful protective system, that we hope will enable millions of people to maintain, and even improve their brain power lifelong.

There are some cautions. The largest is the biochemical and lifestyle differences between individuals. Our records of use of succeeding models of the Brain Program go back for 26 years. But they cover only 1500 or so people, and are taken mostly from fit and healthy folk and from athletes. Although we have not had a single report of toxicity or detrimental side-effects, and much evidence of benefits, from folk who have been on our program for up to two decades, all were given programs individually designed for their personal biochemistry, their medical history, and personal body and lifestyle factors. And they are all under our supervision.

The biochemical and lifestyle individuality of people is so diverse that no one-size-fits-all program can fit everyone, no more than a one-size-fits-all shoe. To attempt to overcome this limitation, I include many ways in which you can individualize strategies to suit your body, your medical history, and your lifestyle. Of course, I have no control over any individual's interpretation or application of the program herein, and all such interpretations and applications are made at your own choice and sole risk.

Most important, no part of Save Your Brain has been approved by the US Food and Drug Administration or by Health Canada. Though we have had several enquiries from government agencies, and I have been engaged from time to time as a consultant to several governments, our work on the brain is not being considered as a health policy by any administration.

Sinner that I am who does not expect forgiveness, I am not a government official, nor a mouthpiece of commerce. If you too are a seeker after truth, then it is given herein to the best of my ability.

And it is referenced properly to the scientific literature, so that you can examine the evidence for yourself, to see whether I have made a good fist of it.

Accepting the above cautions, for people who have not suffered brain damage to the point of incapacity, and for young athletes who have suffered brain damage from the overtraining syndrome, we are firmly convinced that Save Your Brain can reduce such damage. For those who have no apparent decline of the brain, we are convinced that the program can improve normal brain function, and along with it, the function of every tissue and organ in the body. We hope that the average person adopting these strategies becomes smarter, faster, more powerful and graceful in performance, and a lot less subject to the ravages of age. By focusing on the brain in this 21st century, scientists are finally dipping their beakers into the waters of the Fountain of Youth.

Michael Colgan
Saltspring Island
British Columbia
January 2007

Table of Contents

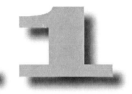

Brain Strain

All along the morning, curdles of cloud knit the sky into sun-honeyed cedars and shoreline pines. Before my window ospreys soar, gulls gab, crows caw, seals surface and dive the duck-bobbing tide, in a land and sea and sky ignorant of artifice. It is the 10th of July 1996, another glorious day at the Colgan Institute retreat on Saltspring Island. As usual, we had fled the heat of San Diego to spend the summer in British Columbia's Gulf Islands, to use the beauty and tranquility to help us solve some of the hard problems besetting our research on aging and human performance.

That year, now more than a decade ago, we were puzzling over two apparently unconnected mysteries: why do healthy adults show measurable declines in mental and physical performance beginning in their mid-thirties, and why do some talented young athletes in their teens and early twenties never recover from the overtraining syndrome and fade into obscurity?

As I watched, the ospreys repeated interlacing circles in the sky again and again, carried effortlessly by the updrafts. It may have been my fancy, but they seemed to trace out a fleeting shape of the mid-sagittal section of the human brain, depicted in Figure 1.1. The common answer to both questions suddenly became clear. Thirty-something adults and former athletes alike are suffering from brain damage.

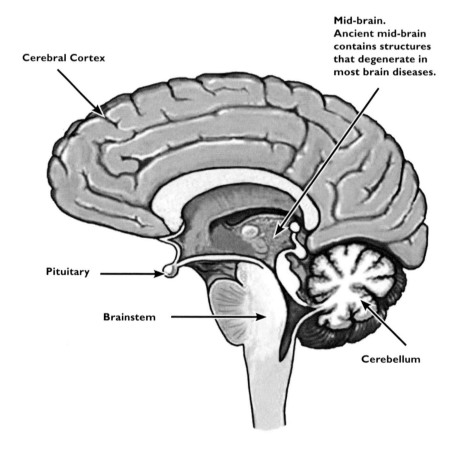

Figure 1.1. Mid-sagittal section of the human brain.

Losing Your Mind

A major discovery from recent research is that most of the brain damage that occurs during usual aging is identical to the brain damage found in all common neurodegenerative diseases.[1] So much so, that many scientists now believe they may be one and the same process. Medical researchers call this process **excitotoxic brain dysfunction**.

By age 35 in most people, the damage becomes measurable as a decline in memory, loss of motor control and balance, and slowing of voluntary movement. By age 60, it becomes noticeable in many people and affects their ability to function in daily life. Finally, on the basis of the predominant symptoms that an individual shows, it is diagnosed as Alzheimer's, Parkinson's, Huntington's, Lou Gehrig's, multiple sclerosis, or one of the many other forms of fatal brain degeneration.[2]

In any individual, the particular symptoms that predominate at the time of diagnosis depend on two factors: the genetic makeup of that individual's brain and the particular traumas and toxins the brain has suffered during life. The genes of some folk make the memory-processing area, called the **hippocampus**, the most vulnerable. As the person ages, it becomes the most damaged area, giving rise to profound loss of short-term memory and a usual diagnosis of Alzheimer's.[3] In other folk, the **dopamine-releasing cells** in the **substantia nigra** become the most damaged, giving rise to tremor and loss of voluntary movement, and a usual diagnosis of Parkinson's.[4] But we know now that both these areas of the brain are being damaged in both diseases, and indeed in almost every one of us from age 35 on.

Brain Disease Is Hardly Inherited

It is still common belief that Alzheimer's, Parkinson's, and other neurodegenerative diseases are primarily familial and unavoidable, caused by defects in genes. Wonderful if you choose the right parents, terrible if you don't. Fortunately, it doesn't work like that. Less than 10% of cases show genetic markers. Even when they are present, the latest research clearly shows that most cases of these genetic defects confer only an increased risk of the disease, **not** the disease itself.[5-9]

This risk is very much like that of folk who inherit fair skin and blue eyes, and who have a higher risk of developing skin cancer than people who inherit darker skin and brown eyes. Whether the lighter-skinned people develop cancer, depends not on their genetic design, but on how much they expose their skin to sunlight. Even in genetically identical twins with a known gene defect for brain disease, the risk of one twin developing the disease if the other twin has it is less than 50%.[6-9] So the major factors that cause the defective gene to express itself and trigger disease have to be environmental.

Michael J. Fox, for example, is a celebrated case of Parkinson's. Because it began when he was a young adult, his illness was considered familial until three other people who worked at the same Canadian television studio in the 1970s also developed Parkinson's. Now researchers are looking for the environmental cause that may lie at that location.

There are many toxic chemicals used in building products and construction today, especially fungicides to inhibit mold. Researchers have documented the "sick building" syndrome for more than 20 years. Fungicides are known to cause disease in office workers, especially in enclosed, artificially-ventilated spaces such as windowless offices and media studios, in which the chemicals are mixed into the air in high concentrations.[10]

Fungicides deserve special mention because we know already that they can cause Parkinson's in farmers. In the small farming community of Fairfield, Montana, for example, because of pesticide exposure, the rate of Parkinson's in older inhabitants is one in every 60 people, compared with the national average of one in about 272, depending on whose figures you take.[11] In a recent representative study, Parkinson's in farmers was linked directly to pesticide exposure, with fungicides being the most likely cause.[12]

These unfortunate people saw no reason to take protective measures against brain disease because the environmental toxin was unsuspected. The latest research has uncovered many of these toxins, and thus offers us strategies to avoid them. Though you cannot choose the genetic makeup you inherit, by correct nutritional and lifestyle choices, you can avoid the environmental triggers that cause defective genes to express themselves and damage your brain.

How Your Brain Gets Damaged

It should be no surprise that brain function starts to decline early in life. Brain cells are more vulnerable than other cells in the body for three main reasons. First, although your brain is less than 2% of your body weight, it uses 20% of your oxygen. So the free radical production in brain cells is many-fold that of other cells. Second, unlike cells in other parts of the body, brain cells are mostly **post-mitotic**, which simply means they are in final form and cannot replicate. So there is no way they can divide and produce clean new cells, and thereby get rid of the choking debris of damage. Third, because they cannot replicate, the loss of brain cells by cell death is permanent.[13]

A dominant cause of the brain damage of usual aging is **free radical** injury to the **mitochondria**, the powerhouses of your cells shown in Figure 1.2. These are the structures that produce the energy that makes you a living being. Free radical damage progressively reduces the ability of mitochondria to make the basic energy molecule, **adenosine triphosphate (ATP)**. So much so, that the average 60-year-old produces only about half the energy of a 20-year old. The resulting decline in the energy supply produces all sorts of mayhem.[13, 14]

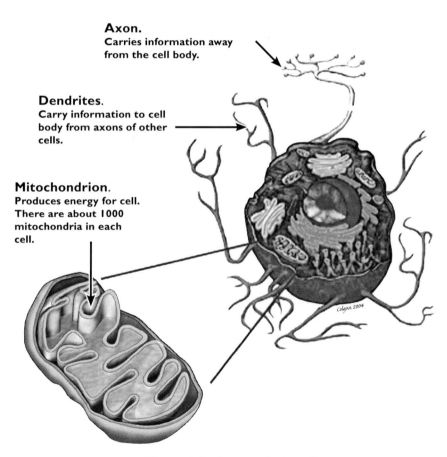

Figure 1.2. A typical brain cell.

Axon.
Carries information away from the cell body.

Dendrites.
Carry information to cell body from axons of other cells.

Mitochondrion.
Produces energy for cell. There are about 1000 mitochondria in each cell.

The Failing Electric Fence

In normal brain function, the mitochondria supply constant electrical energy to provide the power for what are called the **trans-membrane potentials**. These are most easily described as little electric fences around nerve cells that keep damaging substances out of the cell, much like an electric fence keeps cattle out of the wheat field. A decline in energy because of mitochondrial damage causes receptors on nerve cells to lose some of their protective electrical charge. The **glutamate** neurotransmitter system, for example, is responsible for fast, excitatory neural transmission. I will show you how reduced trans-membrane potentials allow excess glutamate to enter and damage specific cell receptors.[15]

You will also learn how the decline in mitochondrial energy disrupts **calcium homeostasis** in the brain. When the electric fence around the cell membrane loses power, calcium leaks into the cell, causing a cascade of damaging events, including a massive increase in free radicals. Accumulation of free radicals from calcium leak (and other causes) damages the DNA which provides the codes for the more than 100,000 different proteins that make up your structure. Progressive errors then creep into the production of proteins that make up your brain.[15]

In addition, free radicals cause fats and proteins in brain cells to oxidize (go rancid), setting up a state of **chronic inflammation**. Some damaged protein fragments also collect in nerve cells and form insoluble **plaque** which inhibits the flow of nerve impulses, much like plaque in arteries inhibits the flow of blood. Free radicals also damage the **microfibrils** of nerve cells, thin tubes that occur in parallel lines like train tracks to facilitate the transport of nutrients and information. Microfibrils also form supporting structures for the cell, similar to steel trusses that hold up a domed building. Free radical damage twists microfibrils into useless **neurofibrillary tangles**, shown in Figure 1.3. They are found most prominently in Alzheimer's disease,[13-15] and resemble strands of wool twisted around each other.

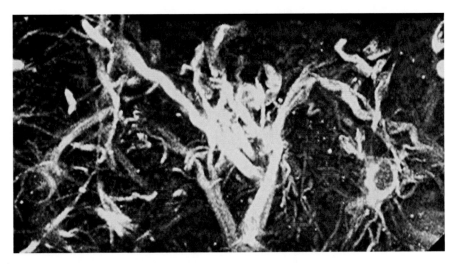

Figure 1.3. Photomicrograph of neurofibrillary tangles in Alzheimer's disease.

We will also cover the essential **nitric oxide** system in the brain, and how it gets out of control and generates the extremely damaging free radical **peroxynitrite**.[15]   And you will learn about **apoptosis**, programmed cell death, an essential brain mechanism which eliminates sick and worn out cells.   When apoptosis goes wild, it attacks the healthy brain cells you need in order to think.[15-18]

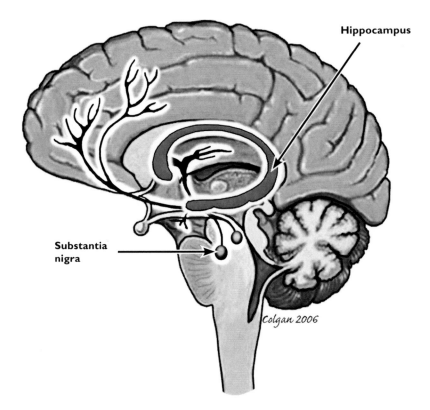

Figure 1.4. Mid-sagital section of the brain showing the hippocampus and the substantia nigra, which are the vulnerable brain structures that degenerate in Alzheimer's and Parkinson's respectively.

Essential **neurotransmitters** in certain areas of the brain also decline with usual aging. Chapters ahead explain how some areas of your mid-brain shown in Figure 1.4 are more vulnerable. The decline of **dopamine** in the **substantia nigra** produces symptoms of Parkinson's, and the decline of **acetylcholine** in the **hippocampus** produces symptoms of Alzheimer's.[16] You will also learn about the types of cell damage happening in all of us that are major gremlins in Lou Gehrig's disease, Huntington's disease, and multiple sclerosis.[17,19]

We know now that many poisons spread throughout the environment by man can trigger brain cell damage and neurotransmitter decline long before the effects of simple aging. Collectively, these poisons are called **zenobiotics**. They include air pollutants, aluminum, lead, pesticides, fungicides, solvents, and tobacco. It is happening to you right now. And now is the time to act to prevent it.

Save Your Brain

You have only a limited number of brain cells that control essential functions, such as memory, motor skills, balance, and reaction speed. The annual rate of loss of these cells determines at what age brain damage will reach the stage of incurable, life-compromising disease. Science now knows these rates of cell loss and has a good handle on ways to reduce them. At the Colgan Institute we do tests of basic brain function to provide individuals with an estimate of the health of their brain and how long they can expect to retain it.

Herein you will learn how to prevent mitochondrial damage and maintain mitochondrial energy production by using combinations of antioxidants and other nutrients that act within brain cells, including **phenyl-butyl-nitrone, R+ lipoic acid**, and **n-acetyl cysteine**. You will learn how we maintain dopamine function in the substantia nigra by using **selegiline**, and acetylcholine function in the hippocampus by using **acetyl-l-carnitine, phosphatidylserine**, and **cytidine-diphosphate choline**.

You will see also how common herbals, such as **silymarin, allicin, genistein, catechins, resveratrol, curcumin**, and **gingko** can exert profound protective effects upon the brain. You will come to know the vital brain roles of **essential fatty acids, carnosine**, and **idebenone**.

I will show you how to avoid brain toxins such as air pollutants, lead, and pesticides. It will take decisive action, but that is the only action which will save your brain. As I write this, Santa Monica beaches have now banned smoking, and the city of Calabasas in California has banned smoking in all public places. Seems draconian now, but remember, it's only a few years since bars, restaurants, and theatres were a fug of smoke.

And you will learn how to program your mind to eliminate the stresses of anxiety, fear and anger that cause extensive brain damage. On the way, I hope we will have a lot of fun.

You Have to Protect Yourself

Current health policies cannot protect you. The massive health benefits and astronomical savings in medical costs that would result from instituting brain protective programs for millions of people who are currently showing only minor symptoms, such as forgetfulness, are beyond the intellectual grasp of current policy makers. Don't be too hard on them. Because of political pressures, many of these folk are concerned only with actions that will benefit their positions while they are in office. Others are old and in poor health, already showing the signs of brain damage and the loss of memory and judgment that are its inevitable consequences.

It will not remain so. I venture to predict that, within 20 years, the strategies outlined here will be considered as important in health policy as vaccination. As study piles upon study, it will become clear beyond ignoring that, if they lose their brains, the aging populations of America and Canada simply cannot stand. Until then, to save your brain from this fate, you have to learn to protect yourself.

The new discoveries that simple nutritional supplements and lifestyle strategies can prevent much of our current epidemic of brain disease will prove a far greater medical advance than the advent of antibiotics. For there is no worse disease than outliving your own intelligence. From the latest research, and our measured and controlled application of it to over 1,500 people, we are convinced that science can not only inhibit the brain damage of usual aging, but can also reverse some damage that has already occurred and can even enhance normal brain function. Many of those who follow our brain program show unmistakable evidence of improved intelligence, memory, and movement, and healthier function in every aspect of their lives.

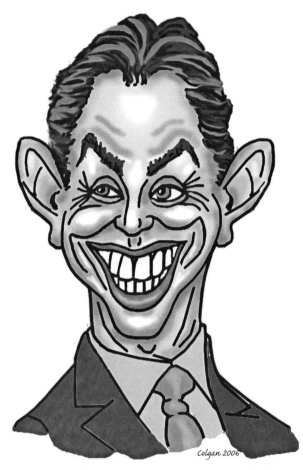

"I know the Mitochondria... full of Extreme Radicals."

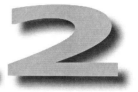

In the Beginning

A cockroach reacts swiftly to light, sound, and smell. It eats, sleeps, runs, and reproduces, but not much else. For these activities, its brain cells work exactly like yours and mine. The neurons or nerve cells that compose the cockroach brain are almost identical to those of the human brain. Our whole genetic plan differs from that of a cockroach by less than 20%. Most of our genome was already formed *before* our evolution diverged from the lineage that led to modern-day bugs. So next time you shudder at one of these odd little scurrying creatures, think for a moment – but for a small divergence in genes, there you run.

The big difference between cockroaches and humans is the complexity of our brain function, which determines the way our bodies function to produce the vast panorama of human behaviors displayed in the dance of life. To understand brain function and how to protect and improve it, we need to take a light-hearted peek at how the brain developed because that is where all the trouble lies.

Evolution of the Brain

Your **central nervous system** consists of the brain and spinal cord. No one really knows how it evolved, so this is a cautionary tale, though based on what evidence we have. We can study its development by following the growth of a baby in the womb (Figure 2.1), and by looking at the fossilized remains of our distant and not-so-distant ancestors.

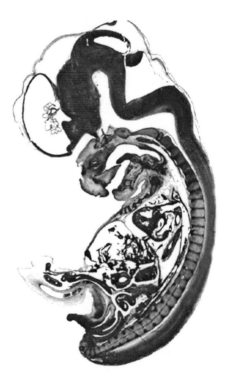

Initially, as with the human fetus today, our ancestors were little more than a tube of nerve cells which animated a surrounding tube of body cells. They lay in the primeval swamps with only one function – reproduction. Then, about 500 million years ago in the Paleozoic era, the nerve cell tube developed

Figure 2.1. Image of human fetus, showing early development of neural tube of brain and spinal cord.

a bump at one end with enough connections to operate a mouth that could suck mud and microscopic creatures for nourishment, passing the debris out the other end. We evolved from this blind, deaf, eel-like creature called ***Amphioxus***, the progeny of which still live on today in the Mediterranean Sea. *Amphioxus* spent its life, hopefully happily, sucking, excreting, and copulating, until these activities wore it out. Meanwhile, it begat new baby tubes to keep the whole peculiar process going.[1]

After a long, long time, a few of these creatures got curious. On the head bump of nerve cells, bits turned outward to have a direct look and sniff at the world, and they grew eyes and a nose. Now they were able to squint out their food more easily. So they had more time off, enough to copulate and to develop the urge to get out of that sucking swamp.

After eons of struggling through the mud, they grew fins on the belly, which eventually became limbs, which enabled them to finally stick their heads up into the sunlight and sniff the fresh air. One of the links between limbed fish and land animals is the coelecanth shown in figure 2.2. It seemed a whole lot nicer than the swamp, so they took up residence on land. But, deprived of protective burrows in the mud, they quickly discovered all manner of predatory creatures who considered their soft, puny bodies a tasty snack. Over many more millions of years, they grew tough reptilian hides, claws, and teeth. And they lengthened their hind legs for running fast, balanced by sticking out their ancient tails. They became **dyapsids**, the progenitors of all mammals. Their brains developed a **limbic system** on top of the original bump of nerve cells, loaded with nuclei that controlled fear, anger, and other prehistoric emotions. Then only the size of a pea, that limbic system became the source of most of our brain disease today. They lived this way for over 100 million years, so the limbic system had plenty of time to become entrenched in our gene pool. It grew and grew.[2]

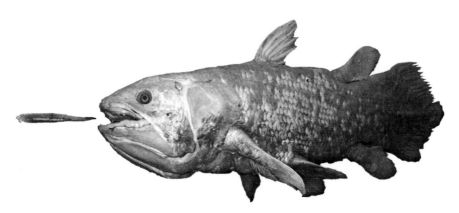

Figure 2.2. Descendents of Amphioxus live on today as the lancelet (left), common in the Mediterranean Sea. After 200 million years, Amphioxus grew fins which eventually lengthened into limbs like those clearly visible on the coelecanth (right), which has existed virtually unchanged for 300 million years. In April 2002, living colonies of coelecanth were filmed off the coast of South Africa.

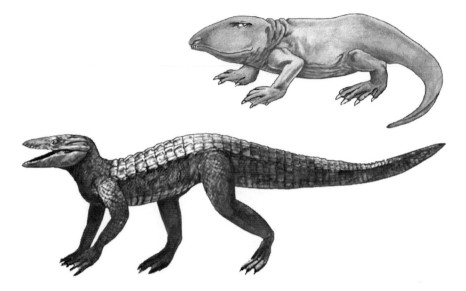

Figure 2.3. In the move from water to land, our fishy ancestors became amphibians with paddle-shaped limbs like those of Eryops (top). They gradually developed into permanent land dwellers called dyapsids (bottom). Brains grew the primitive R-complex of nuclei shown in Figure 2.4, which mediates aggression, fear, and territoriality.

Evolution of Mammals

Some of our distant cousins, however, remained small in brain but grew massive and terrible bodies, such as ***Tyrannosaurus rex***, who could bite through rocks. They made our hearts beat so fast that we began to warm our own bodies independent of the sun. After many more millions of years, we found that the body warmth enabled us to move more swiftly and elude the slowcoach, cold-

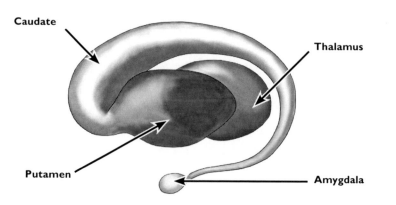

Figure 2.4. The R-complex dominates the brains of reptiles. Buried in the center of human brains, very similar structures shown in Figure 2.5 cause us a lot of emotional trouble and brain dysfunction.

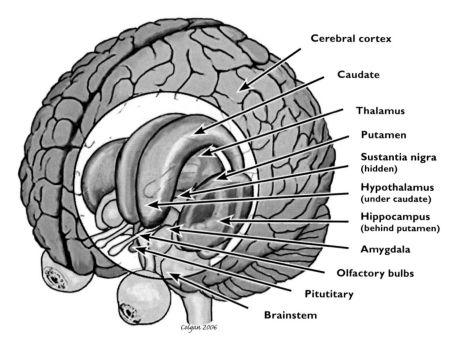

Figure 2.5. The limbic system of the human brain evolved in the early mammals some 60 million years ago. It contains the primary nuclei, inherited from the reptiles, that are involved in all common brain diseases.

blooded dinosaurs. So we replaced our reptilian skin with fur to conserve the heat and resist the cold. And we took refuge from Ty and his friends in tall trees, and grew opposable thumbs to help us climb. After a great while, we could swing nimbly about from long hands and feet, even while eating and copulating. About 50 million years ago we became **prosimians**, some of whom still exist as modern-day lemurs.[3]

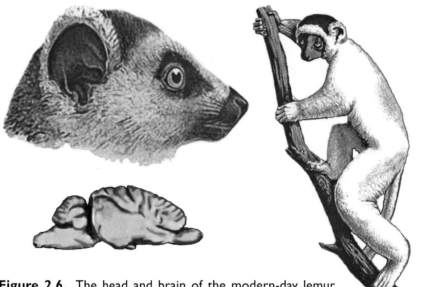

Figure 2.6. The head and brain of the modern-day lemur (left) is very similar to the lemurs from which we likely evolved. Note the large olfactory bulbs and rudimentary cerebral cortex. Painting of lemur (right), adapted from the 1875 edition of *Histoire Physique de Madagascar*. Lemurs still thrive on Madagascar to this day.

Some of us developed further into ape-like creatures who finally shed that vulnerable tail. We were never chimps or monkeys, but did consider them tasty snacks. We began to develop a cerebral cortex on top of the limbic system and the smartest among us became **anthropoids**. Until the last few million years, however, our brains remained small and primitive, our behavior subject to limbic responses to the immediate situation.

About three million years ago, we became, or at least were cousins to, *Australopithecus afarensis* hominids, early progenitors of humanity. Most famous is "Lucy," illustrated in Figure 2.7. She was discovered at Hadar in Ethiopia by Donald Johanson in 1974.[4] With a brain size expanded to 400 cubic centimeters, about one third of our brain size today, the cerebral cortex on top of the limbic system was growing rapidly. The bump in the tube began to think, that is to conduct internal brain activities independent of the immediate surrounding environment.

With this advantage over all other animals, we could reason and plan and quickly became top of the food chain. Lucy stood upright, walked bipedally by swinging her arms, and mused upon her existence. Now we had more time off from eating, cavorting, and copulating than we knew what to do with. So we formed our own special genus, *Homo*, and invented a new game to use up our animal time, blowing air out our intake holes to make complicated weird noises, mostly concerned with who is top tube. *Homo sapiens* is the only animal which developed the brain mechanisms

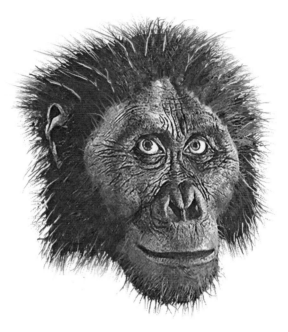

Figure 2.7. This is what "Lucy" may have looked like. **Australopithecus afarensis** hominids, our likely ancestors, lived about three million years ago. New discoveries in 2001 and 2002 suggest that earlier hominids may have existed as far back as seven million years ago.

necessary to learn this trick of abstract communication. Language was born.

After another long while, we realized that the language noises could reach beyond other tubes within earshot, by converting them to squiggles on papyrus leaves, tree bark and rocks, and sticking them up all over the place. Now tubes passing by could see who was top tube, even when we were not there, even when we were dead and gone.[5]

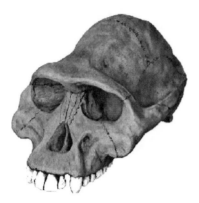 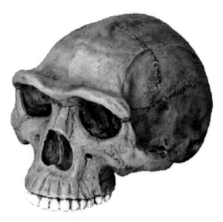

"Lucy." Brain size 400 cc   *Homo erectus.* **Brain size 800 cc**

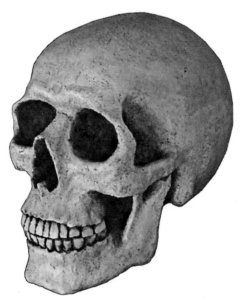

Modern man. Brain size 1200 cc

Figure 2.8. Comparative brain sizes of "Lucy" (top left), an 800,000-year-old *Homo erectus* (top right) and modern-day *Homo sapiens* (bottom). Note upward growth of the skull to accomodate the growing cerebral cortex. (Fossil skulls are reconstructions.)

Thinking of squiggles and trying to remember them forced our cerebral cortex to grow rapidly. Thus, as the evidence suggests, that little clump of nerve cells lying in the swamp developed into the human brain, which spends much of its lifetime today, poring over squiggles on bits of plant fiber made into thin and uniformly rectangular paper, and the fleeting squiggles on computer screens.

But no matter how much we posture on our humanity, make no mistake, we are still classified as animals; class: mammal; order: primate; family: hominidae; genus: homo; species: (we hope) sapiens. Every aspect of our bodies, from the temporary gills of the human fetus to the fingernail remnants of our claws and the vestigial tail on our sacrum, betrays our origins. All the history of the brain is built into our genes. Our brain structure and function reflects that history, and we still think and move to the beat of the primeval.[6]

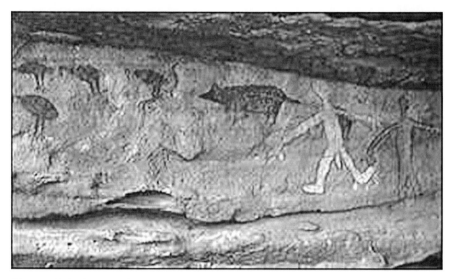

Figure 2.9. Some of the earliest of human squiggles. These rock drawings were found in Lusaka, Zambia, in May 2000, and have been dated to approximately 35,000 years ago.

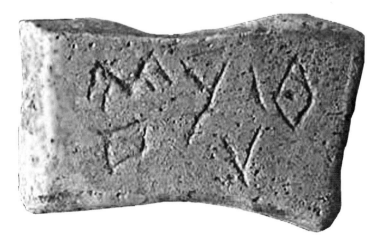

Figure 2.10. Some of the earliest writing. This pottery shard, which is approximately 5,500 years old, was found in 1999 at Harappa in Pakistan, at a site of the ancient Indus civilization.

Thinking Human

I hope that folk of religious conviction can accept this sketch of the evolution of the human brain. To my mind, it does not conflict in any way with the biblical view that God created man in his own image.

> *Made in the image of God personally and purposefully.*
> Genesis, 1:26,2:7

The evolutionary record is undeniable. But all that science has discovered may have been simply steps in a divine plan. If anything, we should consider ourselves privileged that we have been allowed to glimpse the way in which the miracle of life was performed.

And the miracle continues. We are still evolving. We left the swamp, we left the trees. Now we are leaving the Earth entirely. Almost all our squiggles of language today refer to people, places, and events that are not there. They exist only in the effects the squiggles have upon our brains. The language game that we invented to use up our time now controls our lives. We live in our brains, and most of what we conjure there has no existence elsewhere. So we have to be ever alert for the beast rising because there is no limit to what imagination may conjure.

Evidence of our animal limbic system is easy to see. Think of the effects of the word "cancer" on an official medical bit of paper with your name on it. Think of the words "$1,000,000 win" on a missive from the State Lottery Board. The limbic emotions your brain constructs in response to these squiggles can change your life entirely. So you better keep the brain machinery working optimally, to yield the clearest and most powerful thought.

Still unconvinced? Then take the example of millions of otherwise decent German people who were emotionally manipulated by the language of a madman, and set about exterminating millions of equally decent Jewish people for the myth he put in their brains of an "Aryan race." Or the millions of decent Serb and Croat people who had lived in harmony, angered enough to butcher each other for the mental myth of "ethnic cleansing."

As I write these words in July 2006, Israel and Hezbollah, occupying ancient areas of what is called "the Fertile Crescent" where some of the first *Homo sapiens* lived over 100,000 years ago, are at war, each people intent on annihilating the other. In other parts of the Fertile Crescent, Iraqis are intent on killing each other in the most savage manner possible, and others bide their time, intent on destroying whole civilizations if they get the chance. I am sure, gentle reader, that you want your brain to work a bit better than that.

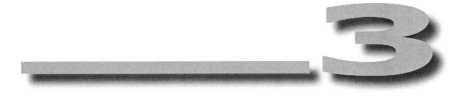

Brains at Risk

Slicing the human brain in half, straight down between the eyes, produces the mid-saggital section shown in Figure 3.1. It reveals a lot about our evolutionary history and the ways in which the brain is likely to degenerate. We start, as evolution did, from the bottom up.

The **brainstem**, consisting of the **pons** and the **medulla**, is the original clump of nerve cells that formed the whole brain of the primitive creatures that began us. As we saw in Chapter 2, this sort of brain still exists today in the blind eel, the lancelet. The most primitive part, the medulla, started as a control system for sucking food in one end and eliminating the debris at the other, plus gag, cough, and sneeze reflexes to get unwanted stuff out the front end in a hurry. The pons came later, when hearts and lungs evolved, to control heartbeat and breathing. The brainstem still mediates these housekeeping functions in us today.

The next step up, the ancient **cerebellum** mediates balance, posture, and automatic and well-learned movements. Sitting on top of our brainstem and forward of the cerebellum is the group of structures which first evolved in the **reptilian brain.** As we saw in Chapter 2, this system existed in our reptilian ancestors 200 million years ago, when they first crawled out of the primeval swamps. This early part of what is loosely called the **limbic system** mediates fear, anger, sexuality, aggression, and territoriality, about the sum total of behaviors that the crocodile is capable of today.[1] It does the same jobs for us.

Above and surrounding the reptilian brain is the later development of the limbic system. These structures developed in the first mammals about 60 million years ago. They are mainly concerned with the sensations we feel in emotions and appetites, including joy and sadness, love and hate, hope and despair, hunger, satiety and sexuality. The content of consciousness we attach to, and use to modify, each of these sensations is much more complex and involves the whole cerebral cortex as well. Without the germ of these sensations in the brains of primitive mammals, we would never have evolved.[1]

To prevent this book becoming a technical nightmare of brain anatomy, in somewhat cavalier fashion, I will limit discussion to the main bits that cause us all the trouble in the excitotoxic degeneration of the brain with age. The ancient structures most involved are shown in Figure 3.1. Their major functions are listed in Table 3.1.

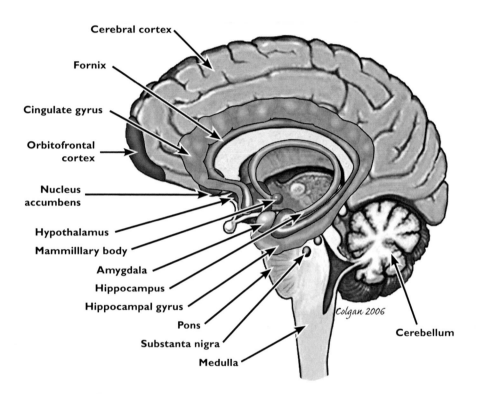

Figure 3.1. Mid-sagittal section through human brain, with limbic system of missing half shown as overlay.

Table 3.1. Parts of the Brain and Their Major Functions	
Amygdala	Involved in systems that mediate aggression, fear, and anxiety.
Hippocampus	Essential for formation of memories; degeneration of the hippocampus is the main cause of Alzheimer's disease.
Hippocampal gyrus	Involved in formation of spatial memories; the hippocampal gyrus degenerates in Alzheimer's disease.
Mammillary body	Important for memory; the mammillary body is structurally abnormal in autism and in old age.
Fornix	Connects the hippocampus to the hypothalamus and mammillary body.
Nucleus accumbens	Involved in feelings of pleasure and comfort; the nucleus accumbens degenerates in cocaine and amphetamine addiction, and in old age.
Hypothalamus	Regulates autonomic functions such as blood pressure and heart rate; controls hormone cascade from the pituitary; regulates hunger, thirst, satiety, sexual arousal, and the sleep/wake cycle; the hypothalmus is involved in pleasure and pain.
Cingulate gyrus	Involved in autonomic functions; essential for attention and cognitive processing; the cingulate gyrus degenerates in Alzheimer's and Parkinson's.
Substantia nigra	Essential for motor movement and balance; degeneration of the substantia nigra with age is the main cause of Parkinson's disease.
Orbitofrontal cortex	Essential for decision making; the orbitofrontal cortex degenerates in Parkinson's disease.

The Keys To Brain Disease

The most important structure in human brain disease is the **hippocampus** of the limbic system, a vital intermediate processing area for learning and memory. The name stems from "hippo," the Greek term for seahorse, the creature whose shape it resembles. The hippocampus, shown in Figure 3.2 in its approximate position inside the brain, is a pair of structures which curl from the temporal lobes of the brain, located above and in front of your ears, to the limbic area in the midbrain. As we will see ahead, damage to these structures is the primary cause of the most prevalent brain disease on Earth – Alzheimer's.

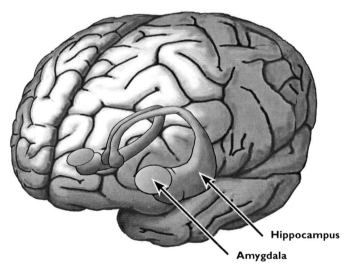

Hippocampus

Amygdala

Figure 3.2. Hippocampus in approximate position as it occurs inside the brain.

Second in importance for brain disease is the substantia nigra ("black body"), shown in Figure 3.3, which is vital for processing motor movement and balance. Buried in the hindbrain deep under the limbic system, this twin structure has many projections to the central limbic area and the **frontal lobes** of the cerebral cortex. It probably existed in the dinosaurs, and likely evolved to enable them to learn to balance and run – fast. But not much else, because they didn't have a cerebral cortex. Damage to the substantia nigra is the primary cause of the second most prevalent brain disease – Parkinson's.

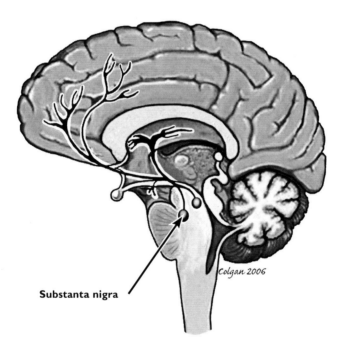

Substanta nigra

Figure 3.3. Substantia nigra shown with its projections to the limbic system and frontal cortex.

Third in importance is the **amygdala**, situated just off the outer end of the hippocampus (see Figure 3.2) which mediates our feelings of fear, hate, anger, anxiety, and panic. This ancient reptilian structure is the target of most anti-anxiety medications but, because it is connected to many complex circuits, the drugs don't work too well. In the human brain, the amygdala is also linked to manic/depressive disorders and obsessive/compulsive behaviors.

Fourth in importance is the **hypothalamus** of the limbic system, shown in Figure 3.4, a set of midline nuclei involved in all of the above aspects of human cognition, plus regulation of hunger, thirst, satiety, and sexual arousal, plus positive feelings such as joy,

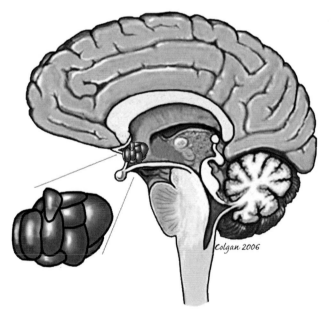

Figure 3.4. Hypothalamus

elation, love, and compassion. It also controls of the flow of brain hormones from the pituitary gland. The hypothalamus even uses the light entering our eyes, to signal the pineal gland to release the hormone melatonin, the synchronizer of the circadian rhythm of our 24-hour sleep/wake cycle, and the daily and seasonal cycles of our whole hormone cascade.

Localization of Brain Function

Note that I have used the words "mediate" and "processing" to describe how the limbic system affects cognition. Largely from the brilliant work of Hans Selye and later Paul MacLean and his colleagues, we have been able to link aspects of our brain function and our consciousness to these structures.[1] But we also know from the same research that particular emotions and traits are ***not*** localized in discrete structures, but are the end result of widespread neural activity throughout the brain.

I am stressing this point because the false idea that discrete brain areas house specific emotions and behaviors is still widely believed. This notion, called **phrenology**, was invented by Austrian anatomist Francis Gall in the early 19th century (Figure 3.5). He theorized that particular emotions and traits were contained in discrete brain "organs", which grew in size from inherited genetic codes to cause specific bumps on the skull.[2] The bigger the bump, the bigger the "organ", and the more that trait affected behavior.

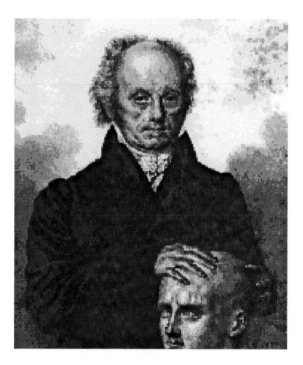

Figure 3.5. Francis Gall, inventor of phrenology

Gall's four-volume, *Anatomy and Physiology of the Nervous System* (1810-1820) written with his pupil Joseph Spurzheim, swept through medicine.[2] Throughout the nineteenth and early twentieth centuries, phrenology became so dominant that a favorite pastime of Victorian gentry was to "have their bumps read." The Victorian phrenology bust in Figure 3.6 shows one of the schemes of localization of each particular trait, suitably refined so as not to offend the ladies of that time.

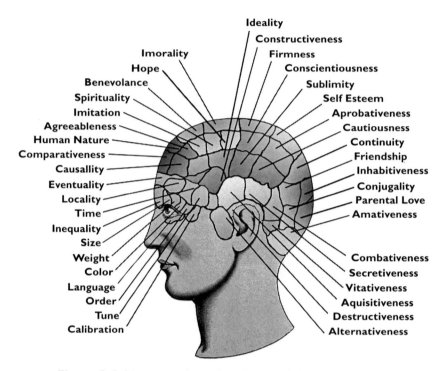

Figure 3.6. Victorian phrenology bust, with knowledge bumps suitably re-named so as not to offend evening soirée sensibilities.

In medicine, interpretation of the bumps was not so tasteful. Many top intellects believed in phrenology as an infallible, unchangeable guide to character, including Emerson and Edison. The revered Boston Medical Society, even believed in skull bumps for "love," "benevolence," and "self-esteem." And woe betide you if you didn't have them, but exhibited the specific bumps for "murder" and "theft" instead.

The *American Phrenological Journal* was published from 1838-1911. It was ve-r-r-ry important. Luminaries, scholars, celebrities, and politicians based their decisions about others and themselves on an individual's "reading". Even in the 1930s, the **psychograph machine**, shown in figure 3.7, was used to give an automatic reading of skull bumps, complete with a printout of dominant traits. These "personality reports" were used to predict important life choices such as suitability of partners for marriage, education, and job promotions.[3,4] A typical pronouncement from the psychograph:

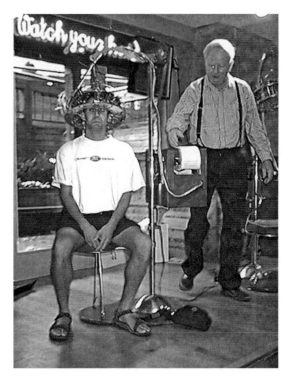

Figure 3.7. Psychograph machine used until 1937 to give phrenological "readings."

"would make a good Zeppelin pilot." About 1935, scientists finally convinced folk that the whole sorry business was a charade, and phrenology promptly departed shamefaced from medicine and languished in the penny arcades.

The notion that brain function, emotions, and character could be predicted from the shape of the skull seems ludicrous now, but we are no more intelligent than the people of Victorian times, and just as liable to fall into the same trap of over-generalization from our medical theories today.

The current fad of predicting future brain disease from discrete genetic markers, as a prelude to cloned replacement brain cells, provides a graphic illustration that modern medicine is not immune from poppycock. So, if at times I seem to boldly go where no scientist ever should, it is in order to make plain statements in a very limited space. As always, I urge the reader to check the references given, to decide whether my judgment is sound.

The influence of phrenology is still very much with us. As an example, Figure 3.8 shows America's most famous poet, Walt Whitman. He was a staunch believer. His writings are widely respected and followed today. He wrote the immortal words of Leaves of Grass based on the principles of phrenology. His own personal "reading" described him as "Christ like." His poem entitled Faces comes directly from Gall's work. His widely used advice on child rearing in the poem, "There was a child went forth",

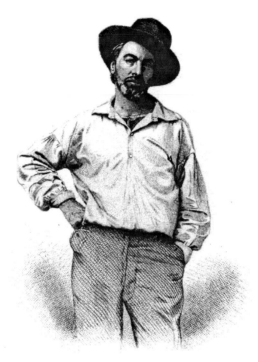

Figure 3.8. Walt Whitman wrote Leaves of Grass following his phrenological beliefs.

reads like a phrenological text.[5]

The Recent Brain

On top of and surrounding the primitive areas of the brain, and composing about two-thirds of its weight, are the right and left hemispheres of the **cerebral cortex**, shown in Figure 3.9. These are the most recently evolved areas, the babies in evolutionary time. The limbic system and lower structures of the brain have been in our gene pool for 60 to 200 million years. The cerebral cortex has been around for only about six million years. The *Homo sapiens* cerebral cortex has been around only about 150,000 years. So it still has a lot to learn.

Yet it is our cerebral cortex that differentiates us from all other animals. It is vital for language, thinking, perception, reasoning, judgment, and other cognitive functions, and for our ability to make precise skilled movements. In most people, language abilities develop mostly in the left hemisphere, visuo-spatial abilities mostly in the right hemisphere.[6]

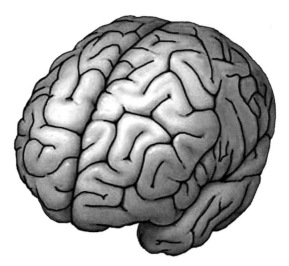

Figure 3.9. Human cerebral cortex.

Control of Thought

A key to understanding brain degeneration, is the clear evidence that the primitive structures of the brainstem and limbic system, that mediate our emotions and appetites, can easily override the recently evolved cerebral cortex that makes us human. These ancient structures evolved in short-lived, primitive creatures, and are not as well designed, nor as robust, as the cerebral cortex. So they are the first brain regions to degenerate under the stresses of our culture and extended lifespan.

A potent example of primitive limbic control of the brain is the overflowing world market for drugs of abuse, including tobacco, alcohol, and most prescription drugs for depression and anxiety. Almost all of these drugs, including heroin, cocaine, opium, and amphetamines, work by affecting limbic structures to produce feelings of pleasure, power, confidence, ease, fear, terror, rage, and panic.[7] Under their influence, messages from the affected structures produce distorted thoughts in the cerebral cortex, ranging from imaginary powers, people, places, and events, to bizarre compulsions to kill and destroy.

The same distortions of thought mark the final stages of the brain damage of usual aging. People suffering brain disease lose communication with the most recent part of our brain design, the cerebral cortex. They revert to more primitive behaviors controlled by the limbic system. That is why they have to spend their last years under heavy medication, both to protect themselves and others, and to support the fleeting remnants of their humanity. A peek at the way in which your brain communicates with itself, and with the world, will help us understand, and hopefully avoid, the same fate.

How You Think

Your brain and body operate by information travelling along nerves. The processing unit that forms the information is the **neuron** or nerve cell depicted in Figure 3.10. A cockroach has about 250,000 neurons. You have more than 100 billion, so many that no one has counted them yet. About three-quarters of the neurons are in your brain and spinal cord, with the bulk in the cerebral cortex, strong evidence that cognition is paramount in the human scheme.

You need some neurons in the body, mainly what are called **afferent** or **sensory neurons** that carry information about the world to your brain. But the vast majority are **efferent** or **motor neurons** in the brain and spinal cord, which carry information out from the brain to activate the body, hopefully in agreement with your thoughts.

Also within the brain are many **interneurons**, by which it communicates with itself. These multiple-connection nerve cells combine and recombine information to produce your consciousness, much like the notes of different instruments in an orchestra combine to produce a Bach concerto. Whether the notes

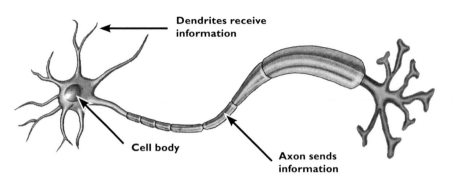

Figure 3.10. Neuron showing axon and dentrites.

of information produce a symphony of wisdom and compassion towards your fellow humans, or a cacophony of homicidal mania, depends largely on the health of the limbic system.

Each neuron has numerous projecting tendrils called **dendrites**, which receive information from adjacent neurons and ferry it to the cell body. The cell then makes a decision to send a signal on or let it die. Signals are sent as an electric current, via a single long tendril called the **axon,** which ferries information to the dendrites of other neurons as much as four feet away. What are popularly called "nerves" in the human body, such as the sciatic nerve, running from your spinal cord to your foot, are simply the long axons of neurons reaching out from the brain and spinal cord, to provide the information necessary to move your arms and legs and sundry other bits.[8]

In the brain, axons from the limbic system run up into the cerebral cortex to stimulate and profoundly influence cognition, memory, and intelligence. They also form the cortical controls of fine motor movement and precise vision, hearing, smell, taste and touch. Incoming signals have to pass through the limbic system before they can reach the cortex. So, when the limbic areas are sick and provide distorted information, as they do in Alzheimer's, Parkinson's and other common brain diseases, the whole brain is sick, too. And the thought that makes us human disappears.

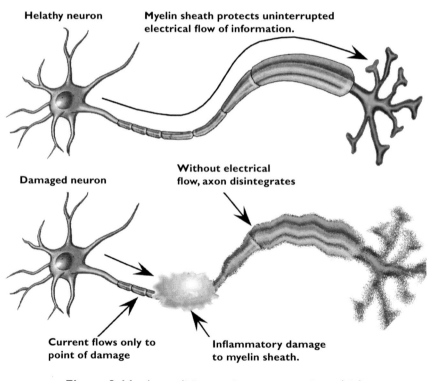

Figure 3.11. Axon disintegration, as occurs in multiple sclerosis and numerous other brain diseases.

Axon Damage

Even when the limbic system is functioning well, and the thought patterns of the cerebral cortex are human and sensible, the brain damage of usual aging may prevent the thoughts from reaching your body in any effective form to activate it. The thoughts have to pass along axons as an electrical signal in order to get to the limbs and organs. That signal is easily interrupted.

The complex and delicate axons are covered with a protective sheath, made of a fatty substance called **myelin**, somewhat like the insulating plastic sheath on an electric cord. When sections of the sheath disintegrate, as they do in the brain damage seen most easily in **multiple sclerosis**, the electrical signal leaks out. The axon is also attacked by body chemicals leaking in. A pocket of inflammation develops, as shown in Figure 3.11. The transmission of information declines. Deprived of its protective myelin sheath and the flow of electrical energy that keeps it healthy, the axon withers and dies.[9]

The Chemical Synapse

In the nervous system of a computer, the circuits are all hard-wired together. As most of us know from weary experience, this design provides a very inflexible means of handling information, less advanced than even the nervous system of a cockroach. Despite all the clever work of Bill Gates, computers remain essentially swift idiots.

Our neurons are not hard-wired. They are separated from each other by little gaps called **synapses**. Within the neuron, information is carried by an electrical signal like that of a computer. But between neurons, the information is carried by chemical means.

Information moves across the synapse, from the axon of each nerve to the dendrites of connecting nerves, by using specific chemical transporters called **neurotransmitters**. These are released from the end bulb of the axon as shown in Figure 3.12. After the information reaches the connecting dendrites, some of the neurotransmitter chemical is broken down by enzymes, and the rest is sucked up into the axon for re-use. This process gives the brain infinite variability

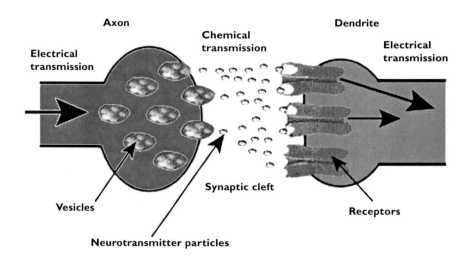

Figure 3.12. Chemical transmission of information across the synapse.

and flexibility in combining and recombining information to produce the symphony of consciousness.[7]

We pay a stiff price for all this brain power. There are numerous different types of neurons, each secreting a dominant chemical neurotransmitter. There are dozens of neurotransmitters plus hormones and helper chemicals involved, inhibiting or complementing each other to impede or facilitate the flow of information. The sum of all these outputs, moment-by-moment, is what we experience as consciousness. Any chemical, environmental, or even emotional input that upsets the chemical balance, can distort your every thought.

In this book we are especially interested in three neurotransmitters in specific areas of the brain. The first is **acetylcholine**, which is vital for memory. We are interested in acetylcholine primarily in the area of the **hippocampus**. The second is **dopamine**, which is vital for voluntary movement and balance, as well as the body's hormone cascade. Dopamine flows primarily from cells in the **substantia nigra**. And the third is **glutamate**, which is an overriding neurotransmitter responsible for fast-excitatory neural transmission.[7]

I should mention here that we will not be addressing the hormones estrogen and testosterone, even though they have strong effects on brain function. The health of the hormone cascade, and effects of hormone decline with aging, is more than a book by itself to even outline the current research. My 1996 book on the subject, *Hormonal Health*, is a useful adjunct to everything herein.[10]

Chemical Distortion

Changing the neurotransmitter mix by putting in even a tiny amount of a chemical that upsets the balance, distorts consciousness. Twenty micrograms of lysergic acid diethylamide (LSD) is so small, you cannot see it on the head of a pin. Yet it disturbs the chemistry of the synapse so violently, that those who use it often see imaginary people and places, or fatally believe they can fly. Repeated use of LSD, if the user survives long enough, permanently damages the brain.[6]

You don't have to risk illicit drugs of abuse to damage your brain. Almost all the prescription drugs for anxiety and depression work by interfering with the chemistry of synapses, primarily in the limbic system.[6] That's why they carry various insert warnings not to operate heavy machinery and suchlike while using them. They alter your emotions and your cognition. Distorted information flows from the limbic system to the cerebral cortex. Judgment and motor skills go out the window.

I applaud Mothers Against Drunk Driving (MADD) for bringing attention to the mayhem caused by the brain effects of alcohol and illicit drugs. But hundreds of thousands of people, on prescription medications that distort their brain, also cause accidents that maim and kill. Yet many of them escape censure because the word "medication" is imbued with a sanctity that courts are reluctant to challenge. If you want to maintain your brain, leave such drugs for the desperate. There are far better ways to tame the beast within.

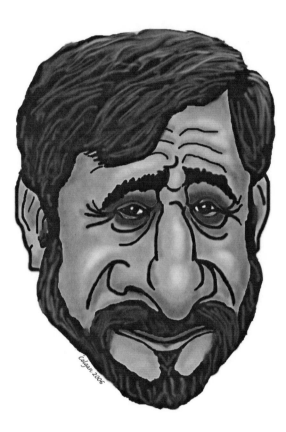

Is this the new face of civilization?

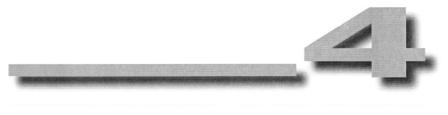

Mitochondrial Decay

Humanity developed by eating plants. This diet included the animals eaten as food too, because they all grow by eating plants. When naturally grown, animals we use for food are simply plants one step removed.

As documented in my book, *Nutrition for Champions*,[1] the battery-bred animal grotesques, which form the bulk of commercial poultry, cattle, pork, and farmed fish today, are plants several steps removed. Often fed on offal until very recently, and still fed on processed garbage grains, they provide inferior nourishment. And the processed pap that lines supermarket shelves is plants numerous steps removed. It provides little nourishment at all. To protect your brain, you should know how closely it is linked to shoots, roots, and leaves. To show you, I have to dismiss a few popular myths.

Plants Are Not Made From Soil

It is common belief that plants grow from the soil and are made mostly of dirt. Any elementary physics text will show you this belief is false. Plants grow very well hydroponically, on no soil at all, using only water containing a tiny smidgeon of dissolved minerals.

When they grow in soil, plants roots seek only the water and mineral mixture. Their structure is composed mostly of nitrogen and carbon dioxide which they extract from the air – plus light. Yes, light, the visible range of the electromagnetic spectrum that is the basic energy force of our universe.

The mixture of minerals and gases, including the gases hydrogen and oxygen that compose their water, permits plant leaves that are spread before the sun to use their green chlorophyll to capture particles of light called photons, as illustrated in Figure 4.1. Some of this light energy is used for growth, but most of it is stored in their structure. All plants, even the largest trees, are storehouses for the energy of the sun. All plants are made mostly of light and gas.[1]

In a tree, the light is concentrated as wood, becoming more and more dense at its core with the force of each annular ring of growth. In ancient buried forests, the light energy is compressed into coal. Early in human history about 1,000,000 years ago, we learned to

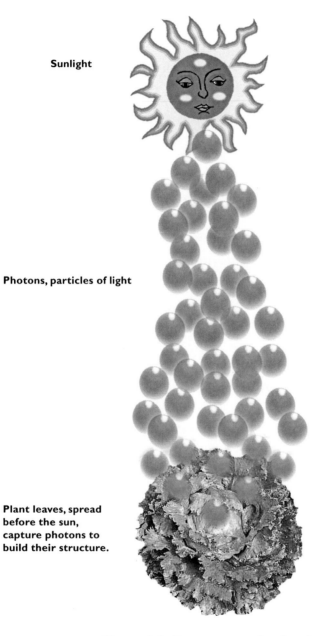

Sunlight

Photons, particles of light

Plant leaves, spread
before the sun,
capture photons to
build their structure.

Figure 4.1. Energy capture by plant foods.

use heat and oxygen to release this energy as fire.[1]

The energy in trees is held too tightly for our weak digestive systems to extract it, which is why we cannot eat wood for nourishment. Other animals, such as deer, cattle, and even porcupines, have stronger digestion and consider wood a tasty snack.

Trees serve us in a different, but equally vital, way. They grow by combining light energy with water and a smidgeon of minerals from the soil, plus air breathed in through small holes on the undersides of their leaves. In this process, they remove and use the carbon dioxide in the air, and return the oxygen as a waste product. The primary reason we should respect the forests is because they maintain the 21% of oxygen in the air that enables our brains to obtain sufficient oxygen.

The suffocating air of crowded cities is more than simply polluted, it is also short of oxygen. Too many people and oxygen-using machines, not enough living green stuff. No surprise that city dwellers often cannot think straight. Their brains are short on gas. There should be good business for lightweight, designer oxygen bottles in urban centers, and oxygen-enhancing air conditioners in high-rises and office buildings, but it hasn't yet caught on. Thought will flow more clearly when it does.

You Are Mainly Light and Gas

In a blade of grass, a sprout of rice, an apple, a cherry, a grape, the light energy is newly caught, lightly held, and easily available to all living creatures. We began to domesticate pleasant-tasting plants of the forests and plains 10,000 years ago, and now call them vegetables, fruits, and grains. When we eat these plants, their store of light energy is transferred to our flesh.

The closer plants are to the state they were in when we evolved the precise bodily mechanisms to utilize them as food, the more effectively they transfer their energy to our bodies. The more processed the plants, whether it be through the gut of a food animal grotesque, or a food-processing factory, the less effective the energy transfer becomes, and the more damaging chemicals it generates. You can take all the smart nutrient supplements you like, but ***unless you base your diet on fresh, organically grown plant foods, you cannot protect your brain.***

Just like plants, our bodies are not composed of dirt either, despite "Ashes to ashes and dust to dust," and all that medieval malarkey. The composition of the human body is shown in Figure 4.2. About 96.5% of you is made of just three gases, hydrogen, oxygen, and nitrogen, plus our carbon base. These four are the most prevalent elements in the Universe, what physicists call CHON.

By eating plants, we absorb a fraction of minerals, but mainly gas and light, held in a mixture of water, carbohydrates, proteins, and fats. Oxygen, the other essential component of our structure, we extract mainly from the air. Just like plants, we too are made mostly of light and gas.

Gasbag is nearer the truth than we like to think. We don't blow about in the wind only because most of our gaseous structure is in the heavy form of water – H_2O, two molecules of hydrogen combined with one molecule of oxygen. We will see ahead how these two gases are critical for the health of the brain.

Carbon	18.5%
Hydrogen	10%
Oxygen	65%
Nitrogen	3%
Total CHON	**96.5%**
Calcium	1.2%
Phosphorus	1.0%
Potassium	0.4%
Sulfur	0.3%
Magnesium	0.1%
All 53 Other Nutrients	0.5%

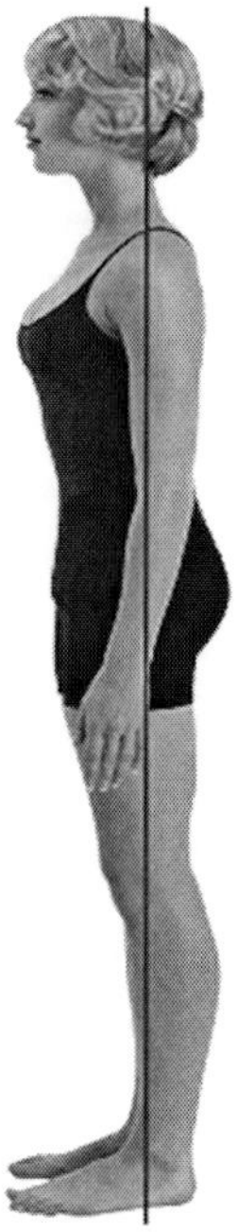

Figure 4.2. Composition of the human body.

The Calorie Myth

One of my favorite myths concerns calories. To keep customers coming back for more, the weight-loss industry holds as a sacred truth that the human body burns food to produce calories of energy. This obsolete notion, still taught to children to keep things simple, is anathema to college teachers like myself who have to undo such learning before they can teach science. The many adults who believe in calories, the continuing emphasis on calories in popular media, and their politically mandated presence on food labels are all warnings that we should be careful what we teach our children. Schoolchild tales become what politicians and the madding crowd believe. To protect your brain, you have to abandon the calorie myth entirely.

Calories are a measure of the heat produced when food is burned in a crude instrument called a bomb calorimeter shown in Figure 4.3. It cannot tell the difference between an apple, which will nourish human life, and a turd which will not. As students, we used to exasperate our professor by burning feces in the calorimeter and solemnly recording their caloric values.

The human body is not a bomb calorimeter. It doesn't "burn" anything. Our flesh is only marginally related to the notion of calories, as anyone who tries to lose weight by counting them quickly discovers. As a young research fellow working in the chronically obese ward at Wellington Hospital in New Zealand 30 years ago,

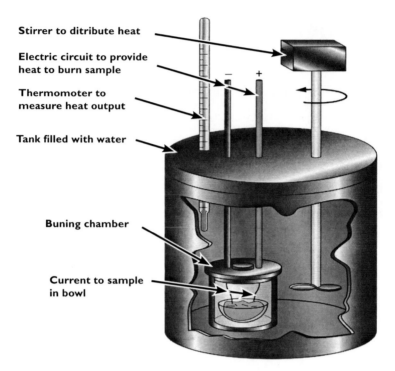

Figure 4.3. Bomb calorimeter

I learned the hard lesson that fat can continue to proliferate on people restricted to a miserable existence of 1,200 calories per day.

Since then science has discovered how to remove excess fat from anyone. With obesity acknowledged as the biggest health problem in Western Society today, it is difficult to understand why this knowledge is not yet official health policy. It was not so long ago, however, that intelligent physicians and health politicians believed in bloodletting and phrenology. Our intellect does not seem to have prospered.

Simply put, the human body works by nuclear power. As outlined in Figure 4.4, the stored energy of sunlight is released from plant foods by a complex process of electron transfer which occurs at the inner membrane of the **mitochondrion**.[2] When you get this process working properly, it requires very little food to maintain a healthy, low-fat body, without hunger and with ample energy for life.

At the nub of life, our soft and feeble flesh releases the infinitely powerful force of the universe – light. In a series of explosive chemical steps, the mitochondria, powerhouses of our cells, extract light energy from food and imprison it temporarily in a fragile chemical cage of **adenosine triphosphate (ATP)**. This volatile cycle is fraught with risk and inevitably damages the brain.

Mitochondria are the most efficient means yet evolved for processing solar energy to power life. But they are not perfect. Humanity is still very much a design in progress. The nuclear function mitochondria perform, variously called **cellular respiration** or the **energy cycle**, is the biggest producer of free radicals in the human body. Approximately 90% of all free radicals in your body are generated right where the energy release occurs, at the inner membrane of the mitochondrion.[1]

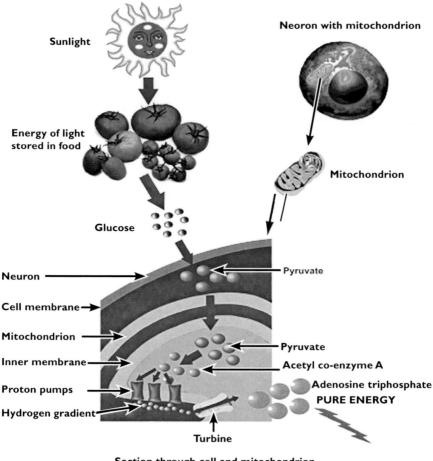

Sunlight

Neoron with mitochondrion

Energy of light stored in food

Mitochondrion

Glucose

Neuron

Pyruvate

Cell membrane

Mitochondrion

Inner membrane

Pyruvate

Acetyl co-enzyme A

Proton pumps

Adenosine triphosphate PURE ENERGY

Hydrogen gradient

Turbine

Section through cell and mitochondrion

Figure 4.4. Formation of ATP and release of energy. Energy cycle for carbohydrates only.

Extracting Energy

Figure 4.5 illustrates how the light energy held in carbohydrates provides some of our energy. To explain, I will briefly describe the simplest process of cellular respiration – the glucose cycle.

Glucose, derived from carbohydrates, passes through the cell wall where it is converted into **pyruvate**. At the outer membrane of the mitochondrion, the pyruvate hands over electrons to transport molecules which then shuttle the electrons into the inner mitochondrial matrix. At the inner mitochondrial membrane, they are converted to **acetyl-coenzyme A**, and the **Krebs cycle** begins. Three proton pumps then move hydrogen ions through the membrane and create a reservoir of hydrogen behind it. Like a hydro dam on a river, the bigger the reservoir, the greater the potential energy. The pressure on the membrane dam forces the

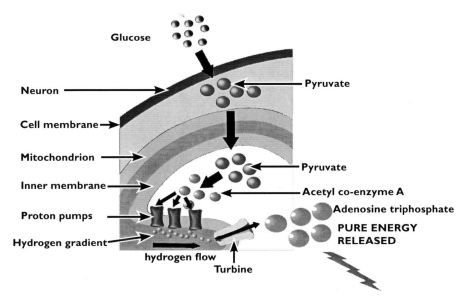

Figure 4.5. Energy release.

hydrogen to flow through the only way out, called **Complex V**, a spinning structure somewhat like a hydro turbine. The turbine makes adenosine triphosphate (ATP).

This process releases the light energy of the universe from carbohydrates and captures it in a simple chemical compound of one molecule of adenosine attached to three molecules of phosphate. The energy is released when ATP fires off one of its phosphates. But how your decision to move an arm or leg causes this release is still way beyond our understanding.

Mitochondrial Damage

Because the mitochondrion is not a perfect machine, about 5% of the energy escapes mitochondrial control and creates **oxygen radicals**. The process of maintaining the reservoir of hydrogen ions also creates waste in the form of **superoxide radicals**. Together these two sources of free radicals progressively damage the mitochondrial membrane.[2]

The membrane dam eventually springs leaks. Hydrogen ions escape through the membrane without going through the turbine and creating ATP. The force in the dam drops, and the energy supply declines. As a result, the mitochondria of people over 60 years of age have lost about 50% of their energy potential.[3] The energy system then has to work a lot harder to keep up the reservoir. So it creates progressively more superoxide radicals, and the cycle of

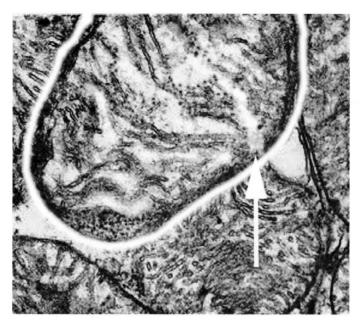

Figure 4.6. Arrow shows damage to mitochondrial inner membrane and leakage (mitochondrion has been outlined in white for clarity).

damage accelerates.[3] With the extreme levels of magnification now possible in electron microscopy, we can directly photograph this damage, as shown in Figure 4.6

Rancidity and Inflammation

Damage occurs not only to the mitochondrial membrane, but also to other proteins and lipids, especially those that make up key enzymes. These particles peroxidize, that is, go rancid. The brain doesn't work too well when bits of it are rancid, even microscopic bits.

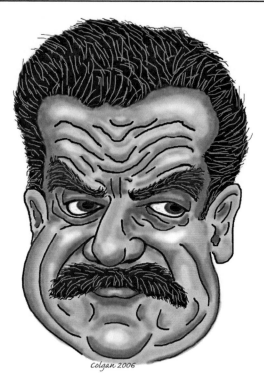

Colgan 2006

Figure 4.7. Example of a chronically inflamed brain.

Equally devastating is the state of **chronic inflammation** which gradually develops in the brain. The substances that control inflammation are called **transcription factors**. A particular molecule we will meet repeatedly is **nuclear factor-kappa B (NF-kappa B)**, a normal part of brain function. Its job is to regulate genetic expression of many inflammatory substances called **cytokines**, a job it does very well. But NF-kappa B is overly sensitive to free radicals. Whenever it is exposed to increased free radicals, it gets furiously overactive. Result – over-expression of cytokines and chronic inflammation of the brain,[4] as depicted in Figure 4.7.

Just like trying to serve with an inflamed tennis elbow, trying to think with an inflamed brain doesn't win a lot of points. Unlike the elbow, however, which gives you gyp each time you swing the racquet, the inflamed brain is silent and unfelt because brain cells have no receptors for pain. So you don't even realize you are thinking like a idiot. Strategies to combat chronic inflammation of the brain are so important that I give them a separate chapter ahead.

Damaged DNA

Free radicals also damage your DNA. To understand the importance of **deoxyribonucleic acid (DNA)**, we need to take a peek at the start of it all. As Stephen Hawking explains most elegantly in his book, *The Universe in a Nutshell*,[5] and John Gribbin describes equally well in his book, *Stardust*,[6] some 15 billion years ago the Big Bang created a Universe full of hydrogen with a smidgeon of helium – and nothing else. The hydrogen formed local concentrations, which eventually became stars, which then transmuted a tiny bit of the hydrogen and helium by nuclear fusion into all the other 100 or so elements that make up everything we know.

Over billions of years, the oldest stars gradually collapsed under their own gravity until the immense pressure caused them to explode into **supernovae** and scatter gas and dust over hundreds of light years of space. Direct photos of a current supernova and a gas cloud from one that occurred many millions of years ago were taken recently by NASA space probes. They are shown in Figures 4.8 and 4.9. This gas and dust mixture then forms new stars. Our sun is one such young star, our planet Earth leftovers of the dusty gas that formed it.

The mass of the Earth today is 29% helium and 70% hydrogen. Everything else totals only 1%. Helium we can leave out of this discussion, as it is an inert gas that does not combine chemically with anything. After hydrogen comes oxygen, the third most common

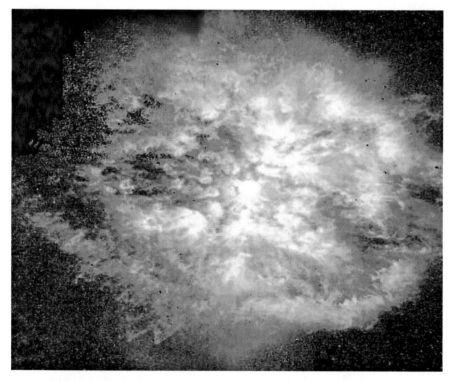

Figure 4.8. Actual supernova (exploding star) tens of light years across (photo composite taken in 2001 by NASA satellite).

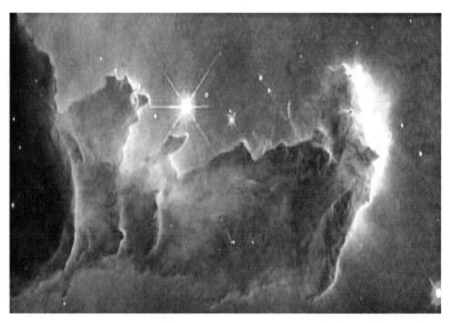

Figure 4.9. Actual dust cloud from an ancient supernova spreading hundreds of light years through the Universe (photo composite taken in 2002 by NASA satellite).

element in the universe. Then comes the fourth, carbon, and the fifth, nitrogen. No surprise then, as we saw earlier in the chapter, 96.5% of the human body is composed of carbon, hydrogen, oxygen, and nitrogen, (CHON) the most common elements in the universe.

Mighty DNA

Fifty-four years ago, on the 28th of February 1953, at the Eagle Pub in Cambridge, England, Francis Crick and James Watson declared:

We have discovered the secret of life.

The real truth about the DNA discovery always deserves mention.

Crick and Watson took the research of Linus Pauling on the nature of the chemical bond (for which Pauling received the 1954 Nobel Prize in Chemistry), plus his almost complete application of that research to cracking the DNA, code which Pauling conceived was a triple helix. They combined this work with the research of Maurice Wilkins who was working at Cambridge on the structure of DNA. They also "acquired," after being refused them, the superb X-ray crystallography images of DNA taken by Rosalind Franklin, as well as her sketches of the double helix.

They rushed it all to print under just their two names before the other owners could take a breath. Even today, few people realize that Wilkins shared the 1962 Nobel Prize in Physiology or Medicine with Crick and Watson for the discovery of the structure of DNA. By then Franklin had died of cancer caused by the X-rays she was using in her research. Nobel Prizes are never awarded posthumously. Nevertheless, by standing on the shoulders of giants, Crick and Watson, neither of whom were trained in chemistry, did manage to work out DNA. Their original signed drawing of the double helix is shown in Figure 4.10.

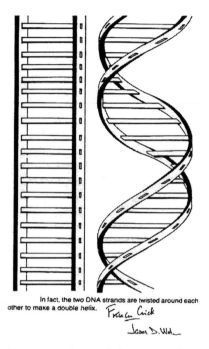

In fact, the two DNA strands are twisted around each
other to make a double helix. *Francis Crick*

James D. Wat___

Figure 4.10. Original signed drawing of the structure of
DNA done by Francis Crick and James Watson in 1953.

The bases of the DNA double helix are four chemicals that are called
nucleotides (see footnote below): **adenine, guanine, thymine**,
and **cytosine**. By combining into millions of different sequences,
these four compose the whole genetic code. They are made entirely
of CHON, that is hydrogen, plus the carbon, oxygen, and nitrogen
created from hydrogen in old stars.[6] The bond that holds the bases

*"Nucleotides" seem to confuse a lot of my students, as the word rarely appears other than in
chemistry texts or in reference to the bases of DNA. There are many nucleotides, the best
known being adenosine triphosphate (ATP), the energy molecule. Nucleotide simply means
a chemical composed of a heterocyclic base (a molecule with at least one ring containing an
atom other than hydrogen), a sugar, and a phosphate group.*

together is also made of hydrogen, the mother element of the universe.

The Hydrogen Bond

This **hydrogen bond**, that is the strength with which hydrogen holds onto other elements, deserves special mention because it is the basis of life. My old mentor, physicist and Nobel Laureate Dick Feynman, was fond of showing in his lectures how all life would wink out if the hydrogen bond failed to let go easily. Unlike the strong bonds made by all other elements, the atomic design of hydrogen makes its bond just weak enough to permit life to occur.

The simplest example is water (H_2O), two molecules of hydrogen linked to one molecule of oxygen. The hydrogen bond holds water together in its liquid form. But when the temperature falls below 4° centigrade, the hydrogen bond releases, enabling the water molecules to move apart from each other to form the crystalline structure of ice. With fewer molecules occupying the same space, ice is lighter than water. So ice floats.

Other liquids all become heavier as they turn solid because their molecules move closer together. With more molecules occupying the same space, their solid form becomes heavier and sinks in their liquid form. If ice did the same, then the oceans would have frozen from the bottom up and life on Earth would never have happened. The unique weak bond of hydrogen gave us the oceans in which we evolved, the remains of which we now carry around as the salty water that fills up our hairy skin bags.

DNA Damage

The hydrogen bond also gave us DNA and the genetic code. Humans have 46 chromosomes (23 pairs), which are chock full of DNA that is tightly wound. When a protein is needed, DNA unwinds and opens up. The hydrogen bond is just sufficient to hold the double helix together, somewhat like the zipper that holds up a dress. This weak link enables the double helix to "unzip," as shown in Figure 4.11. **Ribonucleic acid (RNA)** then jumps in to replicate the DNA pattern, to replace any of the more than 100,000 different proteins required to make up your structure.

Half the dry weight of your body is protein. The structure of all your muscles, bones, and organs is protein. So is your blood, your eyes, your nerves, and all your enzymes. Even your genes are protein, every one.

The codes that define different proteins can have patterns hundreds of bases long, like a very long string of beads. The code for human growth hormone, for example, is 191 amino acids long. If even one of the beads is missing or transposed into the wrong position on the string, the pattern is distorted, the protein made from it is defective, and life is compromised.[9]

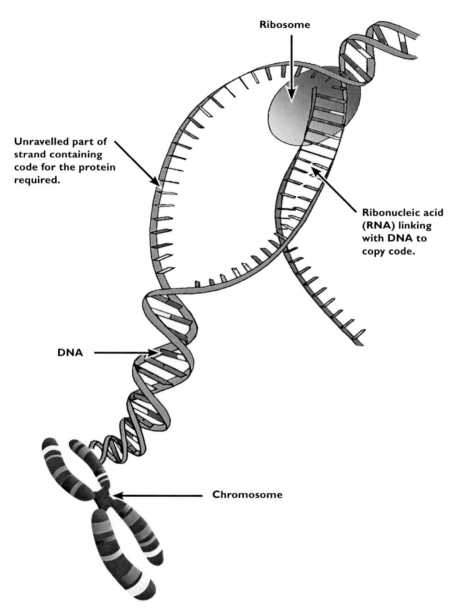

Figure 4.11. DNA opens up, "unzips" from its tightly wound coil in any of your 46 chromosomes to allow RNA to copy the code for a protein.

Recent research confirms that the worst damage to proteins occurs at the inner membrane of the mitochondrion. We now know the details of 15 key proteins that are made there, right alongside the site where energy is released and the nastiest free radicals are formed.[1,7,8] Protecting DNA at the inner membrane of the mitochondrion is a major focus of our **Brain Program**.

I hope this brief sketch is sufficient to convince you that we are composed mainly of gas, plus the infinitely powerful energy force of light. In harnessing the light to animate our flesh, the mitochondria inevitably suffer damage by free radicals. Additionally, free radicals give rise to a state of chronic inflammation in the brain.

We have seen also how the complex DNA code for human life developed over billions of years from hydrogen, the mother substance of the universe, and how this genetic pattern gets damaged. In our efforts to protect mitochondria and DNA, so as to maintain brain function, we are juggling with the origins of everything. No mean task for creatures composed of the debris of stars.

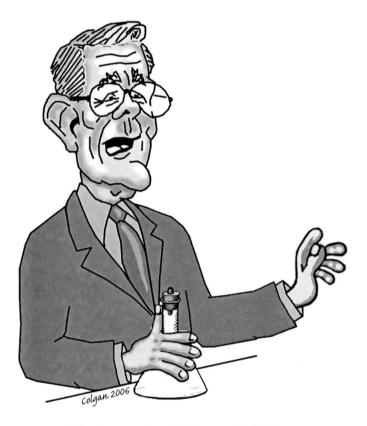

"Nuclear smuclear! We've got his DNA and
we're going to interrogate the hell out of it."

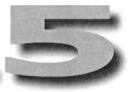

Saving Your Mitochondria

I have reviewed the four main processes of mitochondrial decay. The first is decline in the energy supply, due mainly to continual free radical damage to the mitochondrial membrane. Second is cumulative free radical damage to other lipids and proteins inside the cell, damage that turns them rancid. Third is a state of chronic inflammation of the brain, caused by free radical driven over-expression of the inflammatory cascade. Fourth is free radical damage to mitochondrial DNA, which destroys bits of the genetic code. We are pretty sure from recent research that these processes underlie most of the brain disease that besets humanity, including most of Alzheimer's, Parkinson's, Lou Gehrig's, Huntington's, and multiple sclerosis.[1-5]

Denman Harman first proposed the **free radical theory of aging** in 1954 while working at the Donner Laboratory of the University of California at Berkeley. With extraordinary insight, because there were few supporting data at the time, he reasoned that we age because of oxidation damage, somewhat like the rusting of a steel plate or the gradual crumbling of even granite rock.

When he published the work in 1956, he suggested that any good antioxidant might afford protection and extend human life.[6] Scientists worldwide recognized the importance of Harman's theory and set about eagerly to test it. In thousands of experiments since, the major nutrient antioxidants did protect the heart, circulatory system, and other organs from some oxidation damage, but failed utterly to increase lifespan. Harman seemed to be dead wrong.

In a typical study that tested the nub of the theory, Lee and Hughes at the Institute of Food Research in Norwich, England, repeatedly tested high doses of vitamin C and E for their ability to inhibit two important factors in aging, increased expression of inflammatory cytokines and chronic inflammation within cells. They found no effect on either process of aging damage.[7]

Two decades later, Harman realized that the energy cycle, the process of releasing light energy at the inner membrane of the mitochondrion, is the prime generator of free radicals in the human body, responsible for about 90% of all free radicals. Therefore, the mitochondrion is the structure most vulnerable to aging damage.[8] Meanwhile, however, the whole vitamin supplement industry had seized upon the idea of antioxidants, and made fantasy claims about their ability to prevent aging in order to sell billions of their products, much to the dismay of legitimate scientists.

After many confirming experiments, most scientists have now come to accept Harman's second theory as the fundamental process of the damage of age. It is termed the **mitochondrial free radical theory of aging**.[8] The basic idea is sketched in Figure 5.1. To save your brain and the body that goes with it, you have to learn to save your mitochondria.

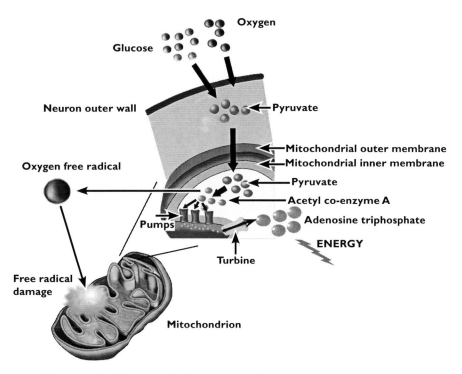

Figure 5.1. Mitochondrial free radical damage, which occurs as part of the energy cycle, is the fundamental process by which we age.

Mitochondrial Antioxidants

As Harman reasoned in 1972, by genius (and serendipity, as it happens), protecting mitochondria requires substances that normally occur *inside* cells and are metabolized there.[8] Mitochondria can be saved only by mitochondrial antioxidants. They are not well known yet, but they will be. It takes a bit of chemistry to get a handle on their action, but it's well worth the effort.

The first mitochondrial antioxidant we will consider is one of the most important, **alpha-lipoic acid**. But it has to be the right alpha-lipoic acid. Many nutrients can be made in two distinct shapes called isomers. One form has what is simply described as a left-hand twist to its molecular structure, the other a right-hand twist. When the two forms are exact mirror images of each other, as is the case with alpha-lipoic acid, they are called **enantiomers**.

Usually, only one enantiomer occurs in Nature. The other is a man-made chemical. We have to be very wary of man-made chemicals because Nature designed all the locks in the human body and holds all the keys. Your body has locks only for those substances that were present on Earth during the time that humanity evolved. They were the substances from which the human genome designed itself.[9] The job took at least 6 million years.[10] Our genetic code has not changed a whit in the last 10,000 years. As Stephen Hawking explains so eloquently, any chemical made by man was never experienced during evolution and is unlikely to fit our design.

The best known example is vitamin E. The ancient, natural isomer that occurred in plant oils is **d-alpha tocopherol**. It has the exact twist to fit human flesh because evolution worked to develop the exact lock for it over millions of years. The synthetic, man-made isomer, **l-alpha tocopherol**, twists the wrong way. It does not fit your flesh and is useless for human nutrition. Worse, it interferes with the action of the natural d-isomer.[9] Most people know not to buy any supplement containing dl-alpha tocopherol, though you still see them on pharmacy shelves, and they are still used by the ignorant, even in some medical studies.

The Right Lipoic Acid

Lipoic acid exists in Nature as the **R+ isomer**. The R+ is the twist that fits your body locks. But most commercial supplements are synthetic. They are what is called a racemate of alpha-lipoic acid. They contain about 50% of R+ lipoic acid and 50% of its mirror image, S- lipoic acid. The S- isomer does not occur in Nature and does not fit your body. Worse, the S- isomer interferes with the R+ isomer and inhibits its action.[11] These kinds of errors occur frequently when our meager commercial chemistry tries to match the complexity of Nature.

In a representative study, researchers exposed nerve cells to a poison called buthionine sulfoxamine that kills cells by inhibiting their antioxidant defenses. R+ lipoic acid reduced cell damage by nearly 50%. The R+S- racemate, still sold in most supplements, had no effect.[12] So how can supplement manufacturers get away with selling the S- form? Don't be too hard on them. Until recently they didn't know any better. This is fairly new science. It is only in the last ten years, that scientists have uncovered the uselessness and potential harm of synthetic S- lipoic acid. New findings often take more than a decade to percolate down to the marketplace.

By the way, only "natural" chemicals can be replaced commercially by man-made racemates without testing to see if the man-made isomer works or not. Long ago, scientists found out that man-made versions of pharmaceutical drugs frequently didn't work at all. Today, by law, both isomers of brand-name drugs have to be rigorously tested, and the formulas adjusted as necessary for maximum effect, before they are permitted to be sold. That's one big reason brand-name pharmaceuticals work, although you cannot place as much confidence in cheap generic knock-offs.

Effects of R+ Lipoic Acid

There are hundreds of studies on R+ lipoic acid, but space permits me to cover only a fraction. I will confine discussion to just one important effect of R+ lipoic acid: it raises the level and activity of the endogenous mitochondrial antioxidant **glutathione**. Glutathione is a vital part of our intracellular defense system against oxygen, without which we would not last more than a year. One reason that humans live so long, is that we evolved a better antioxidant defense system than all other mammals.

Pet dogs provide a familiar example. Perhaps because of many centuries of in-breeding, they have inefficient glutathione defenses, suffer much more oxidation damage to their DNA and mitochondria than we do, and live only 8 – 20 years, depending on breed. If you feed them the right antioxidants and other nutrients, as we do ours at the Colgan Institute, dogs live about 20% longer than the average. They're a lot perkier, too. You can get many more years with your favorite pet if you avoid the TV commercials and feed them what their DNA designed them to eat. Be warned, however, that the right antioxidants will also cause pedigree pets to grow larger than the breed standard, so they will not be accepted in the show ring.

Glutathione is produced inside your cells. It is the body's most effective detoxifier of chemicals, heavy metals, and other pollutants. It modulates the inflammatory cascade, keeping it under control. It regulates the synthesis of proteins. It regulates cellular enzymes. And it repairs DNA. It's a busy molecule.

Trouble is, glutathione declines with age. One big reason is that the human body has no way of getting rid of excess iron. We build up iron in the brain. Through a complicated chemical process, excess iron slowly destroys the glutathione defense system.[13]

Researchers at the State University of Oregon showed recently that R+ lipoic acid given to old subjects, reverses the age-related accumulation of iron and restores glutathione status.[13] In another

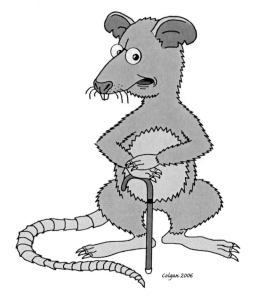

Colgan 2006

"OK, so you made me perky. It's not helping my arthritis."

recent study, Tory Hagen and colleagues at the Linus Pauling Institute, showed that R+ lipoic acid raised the level of glutathione in old rats beyond that of young controls (Figure 5.2). It also made the oldsters very perky, more than doubling their activity levels.[14]

This study is representative of research on R+ lipoic acid. The findings are important for our goal of maintaining and even improving brain function because there is now clear evidence that low levels of glutathione are linked to vascular forms of dementia,[15] Alzheimer's disease,[16] Parkinson's disease,[17] and multiple sclerosis.[18] That's the majority of the brain disease we are trying to prevent. Not many other natural, non-toxic molecules can hold a candle to R+ lipoic acid.

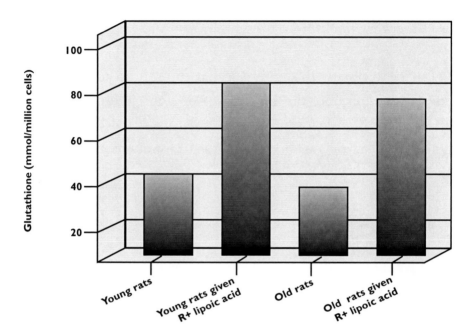

Figure 5.2. R+ lipoic acid raises glutathione levels in old
rats to beyond the level in untreated young rats.[14]

By raising glutathione levels and by independent mechanisms
that we don't understand too well yet, R+ lipoic acid also protects
the retina (part of the brain turned outwards) against diabetic
retinopathy, and protects the retina and your sight against the
degeneration of usual aging.[19, 20]   It even seems to protect the
insulin system against aging and has been proposed for treatment
of adult-onset diabetes.[19-21] Insulin resistance is another key part of
the degeneration of aging that happens to everyone. If you want to
fully protect your brain, you will also have to protect your insulin
system. It is beyond our discussion in this book, but is covered in

two other new books from the Colgan Institute.[10, 22]

My space to discuss R+ lipoic acid has run out, so to bolster my case I want to quote the conclusions of some leading scientists. Lester Packer, head of the Packer Laboratory at the University of California, Berkeley, is the world's most prominent researcher on lipoic acid. In 1999 Dr. Packer stated:

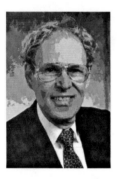

R(+) lipoic acid and not a racemic mixture of R(+) and S(-) lipoic acid should be considered a choice for therapeutic applications.[23]

Renowned researcher on antioxidants, Bruce Ames, Professor of Biochemistry at the University of California Berkeley, is even more definite:

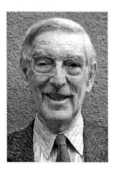

Lipoic acid sold in a health food store is a synthetic mixture, a racemic mixture. And R(+) is the natural form and S(-) is an unnatural form. And in our hands, R(+) works and S(-) doesn't.[24]

The R+S- racemic mixtures will eventually drop out of the marketplace. Meanwhile a few smart companies, who keep up with the science, are using R+ lipoic acid for their supplements. You should, too.

Glutathione

The obvious question that crops up in my lectures is: why not take glutathione itself; why bother about R+ lipoic acid? The answer is pretty simple. Lots of companies will sell you a wide variety of glutathiones, but they will not do you any good. Glutathione in any form, taken by mouth, or injected, cannot pass the blood/brain barrier. It cannot get into your brain.[16]

One important finding has come out of research in this area. A potent precursor of glutathione is the amino acid **cysteine**. Even with R+ lipoic acid, there still may be a need for additional cysteine to fully restore glutathione levels.[25] The best way of providing extra cysteine is to take it by mouth in the form of **n-acetyl cysteine**. Even as a supplement by itself, n-acetyl cysteine raises glutathione levels and reduces both mitochondrial damage and DNA damage.[26]

Acetyl-l-Carnitine

Acetyl-l-carnitine is another mitochondrial metabolite important to our brain program. It is proven to increase ATP production.[24] As we noted in earlier chapters, between the ages of 20 and 60,

ATP production in human brain cells declines on average by 50%, causing all sorts of mayhem. Acetyl-l-carnitine is also a substrate for the neurotransmitter acetylcholine, which chapters ahead will show you is crucial for memory.[27] But when you combine acetyl-l-carnitine with R+ lipoic acid, it really shines.

In April 2002, Bruce Ames and colleagues at the University of California, Berkeley, reviewed their recent studies with rats. Acetyl-l-carnitine plus R+ lipoic acid fed to aged rats, reduces the damage to brain lipids and proteins, protects the mitochondria from brain toxins, delays the aging of cells, and protects neurons from free radicals. More important for the delay in brain aging that we are seeking, these two nutrients combined also improve memory, and motor movement.[28] That's an impressive list.

Other recent reports from the same group, and from Tory Hagen and colleagues at the Linus Pauling Institute of Oregon State University, confirm that the two nutrients combined have synergistic action. In one recent study, acetyl-l-carnitine plus R+ lipoic acid reversed mitochondrial decay in aged rats. Both spatial and temporal memory improved far more than with either nutrient alone.[1]

In a second study comparing old and young rats, acetyl-l-carnitine plus R+ lipoic acid improved mitochondrial function and motor movement to a much greater extent in the old rats. Some degenerative aspects of aging were restored to levels found in the young rats.[29]

These and similar studies indicate that acetyl-l-carnitine should be used always in combination with R+ lipoic acid.

There are many other beneficial effects of acetyl-l-carnitine that are way beyond the confines of this brief book, but I want to mention one other recent advance in the research that has big implications for our brain program. It concerns **cardiolipin**. This phospholipid (phosphorus and fat compound) is composed of four unsaturated fatty acids. (These fatty acids are derived continuously from the essential fats you eat, a topic covered in my new book, *Nutrition for Champions*. We will return to them later herein, as you cannot be healthy without essential fats. Cardiolipin makes up about 20% of the structure of the mitochondrial membrane. It is essential

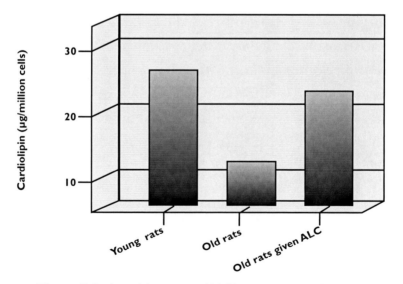

Figure 5.3. Acetyl-l-carnitine (ALC) restores mitochondrial membrane cardiolipin levels to that of young animals.

to stabilize the electron transport chain in the energy cycle that we examined in previous chapters, the mitochondrial part of which is shown in Figure 5.1. It is also essential for apoptosis, the orderly removal of defective, dying, and worn-out mitochondria. Cardiolipin is a big player in the health of your brain cells.

With usual aging, even with all the other supplements you can think of, cardiolipin disappears like smoke, and all the functions it supports decline.[30] The good news is that acetyl-l-carnitine, given by mouth in animal studies, restores cardiolipin in aged animals almost to levels found in the young[31] (Figure 5.3).

Idebenone

Co-enzyme Q10 is sometimes called the "mitochondrial nutrient" because it is involved not only in neutralizing free radicals, but also in transporting electrons into the mitochondria for ATP production. But the development of **idebenone**, an analog of CoQ10, by Imre Zs Nagy of the University Medical School in Debrecen, Hungary, has left the parent in the dust. Taken by mouth, idebenone slips through the blood/brain barrier like an eel.[32]

In cultured cortical neurons, idebenone prevents damage caused by deliberately introduced toxins.[33] It is also being used successfully in treatment of **MELAS disease** (mitochondrial myopathy, encephalopathy, lactic acidosis, and stroke).[33] Further, idebenone has become a treatment of choice in the mitochondrial myopathy of the heart that is part of the brain disease called **Friedreich's ataxia**.[34]

Idebenone also shows promise for Alzheimer's. In studies with rats, infusion with beta-amyloid plaque, of the kind found in the brains of Alzheimer's patients, severely impairs learning and spatial memory. Pre-treatment with idebenone, given by mouth, prevents most of the impairment.[35]

In human trials, idebenone was recently compared with the Alzheimer's prescription drug **tacrine** in a large multi-center, 60-week study. Alzheimer's patients receiving 360 mg of idebenone per day showed greater improvement in cognitive function and daily living activities than those receiving tacrine.[36] These and similar studies indicate that idebenone is an important development for protection of the brain. Non-toxic up to 400 mg per day, it forms an integral part of our brain program.

Selegiline

We have used **selegiline** (Deprenyl, Jumex, Selepryl) at the Colgan Institute since 1985, both to inhibit the age-related decline in the neurotransmitter dopamine, and to prevent the death of dopamine-producing cells in the substantia nigra of the brain, death which leads to Parkinson's disease. As I have documented elsewhere, it works very well.[27]

Selegiline used to be sold over-the-counter in the US. But in 1989, it was approved by the FDA as an adjunctive treatment for Parkinson's disease because clinical trials showed that it significantly increases survival time. It then became a prescription drug and, of course, much more expensive. Whatever the price of selegiline, it is well worth paying to save your brain.

Selegiline is a potent inhibitor of **monoamine oxidase-B (MAO-B)**, a vital regulator of the neurotransmitter dopamine. MAO-B breaks down dopamine and protects brain cells from dopamine overload. If you take too much selegiline, dopamine runs out of control and damages brain cells. Because of this problem some physicians will not recommend selegiline at all.

They are mistaken. Numerous studies show that dopamine declines with usual aging, with consequential declines in brain function and in your hormone cascade from the pituitary gland, which is also largely under dopamine control.[27] Judicious use of selegiline to maintain dopamine function is, therefore, a potent protective strategy for the brain. The main way selegiline works is shown in Figure 5.4.

New research shows that selegiline has even more potent benefits than we realized. These benefits are independent of its effects on MAO-B. We know now that pretreatment of animals with selegiline protects all four of the major classes of brain neurons – dopaminergic, cholinergic, adrenergic and seritoninergic

– from a variety of brain poisons. These include the very nasty, **methyl-phenyl-tetrahydropyridine (MPTP)**, which is used in experimental studies to deliberately damage brains of animals.[37]

Selegiline also reduces free radical production, up-regulates the endogenous cellular antioxidants **superoxide dismutase** and **catalase**, and blocks toxin-induced damage to the mitochondrial membrane.[37]

Finally, and completely unrelated to its MAO-B inhibition,

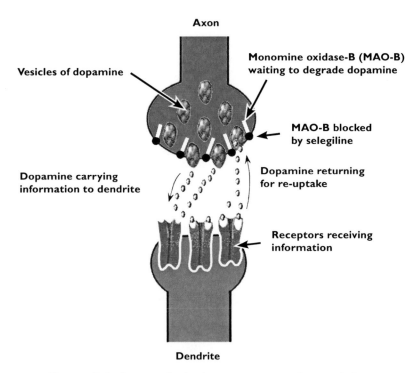

Figure 5.4. Action of selegiline in increasing dopamine function.

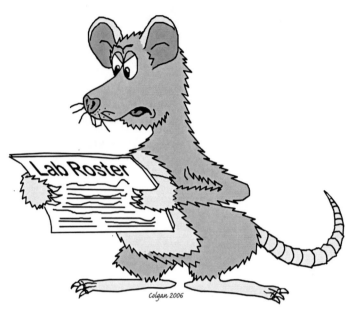

"Wait a minute. I didn't sign up for this!"

selegiline inhibits the free radical production that naturally occurs with dopamine use by the brain.[38] Clinical trials with animals, with healthy people, and with Alzheimer's patients show that selegiline also improves cognition.[39] It forms part of every brain program we undertake.

Selegiline Dosage

The world expert on selegiline is the man who developed it, Joseph Knoll of Semmelweis University in Hungary. As Knoll documents, doses of 1–6 mg per day, depending on age, are sufficient to maintain the dopamine system.[40] Within this range, selegiline has no known side-effects. Above 10 mg per day, however, you are in risky territory. Above 20 mg per day, selegiline is definitely toxic,[41] as some young athletes have discovered when vainly trying to use it to enhance performance. It doesn't, by the way. The dosages we use are given in the table below.

Table 5.1. Colgan Institute Use of Selegiline

Biological Age*	Males (mg/day)	Females(mg/day)
30 – 35	1.0	0.5
36 – 40	1.5	1.0
41 – 45	2.0	1.5
46 – 50	3.0	2.5
51 – 55	4.0	3.0
56 – 60	5.0	4.0
Beyond 60	6.0	5.0

*Biological age is calculated from the Colgan Biomarkers of Aging Scale. These tests are performed at the Colgan Institute as part of our two-day Nutrition and Performance Assessment.
In contrast to chronological age (time since birth), biological age is a composite of scores achieved on biomarker tests of aging in reference to the average scores at different chronological ages in the general population. Biological age can be greater than chronological age in individuals who have aged at a faster than average rate, less than chronological age in individuals who have aged more slowly.

CDP Choline

Phosphatidylcholine is a phospholipid, that is, a combination of the mineral phosphorus and fat. It is a vital component of nerve cell membranes, a component that declines with usual aging.[42] It is also an essential precursor of the neurotransmitter acetylcholine, intimately involved in memory.[43]

Phosphatidylcholine became a popular supplement in the 1980s when numerous studies tried it with Alzheimer's patients in attempts to restore memory. They were unsuccessful. Intact phosphatidylcholine has great difficulty passing through the blood/brain barrier and getting into brain cells.[43]

Recent research shows that oral supplements of some precursors of acetylcholine, namely, **phosphatidylserine** and **citicholine** get into the brain very nicely. Here we will focus on citicholine, as it also serves as a precursor for phosphatidylserine in the brain.[44] So, hopefully, we can get the job done with only one nutrient.

Citicholine is more properly called **CDP choline**, that is, **cytidine 5'-diphosphate choline**. It has at least four strong effects. First, in animal studies, oral supplementation with CDP-choline raises levels of phosphatidylcholine in brain cell membranes, including mitochondrial membranes.[44] Second, CDP-choline inhibits lipid peroxidation, that is, prevents some fats going rancid. Third, it helps protect the essential component of the inner mitochondrial membrane, cardiolipin, discussed earlier in this chapter. Fourth, it stimulates production of the endogenous antioxidant glutathione.[45]

Equally important, but not specific to mitochondria, CDP choline increases production and availability of the neurotransmitter acetylcholine.[43] It bears repeating that decline of acetylcholine is part of the brain damage of usual aging, the main cause of the loss of memory function that finally manifests as Alzheimer's.

With these proven effects, you might expect CDP choline to show benefits in brain disease. Recent clinical trials with older healthy people and with *early* Alzheimer's patients show that this natural substance dramatically improves failing memory.[29,30]

The word "early" is crucial. Trials with animals who are deprived of oxygen to the brain show that pre-treatment with CDP-choline provides significant protection.[46] Giving CDP choline after the oxygen deprivation has damaged the brain has little effect.

That's why it doesn't work too well in cardiovascular trauma. When CDP-choline is used against stroke, as it is in Europe and Japan, it can only be given as a treatment *after* the stroke has occurred. By then many brain cells are dead and beyond help. So is much of the microcirculation to the injured area. Nothing can help dead cells.

It is a very similar picture in a brain that has suffered significant damage with aging. The CDP-choline has great difficulty reaching the injured areas because the blood supply is diminished. And if it does get there, it cannot bring dead cells back to life. So the benefits are small.[47] That is the problem with *all* the current treatments of brain disease in Western Society. Too little, too late. The time to begin using CDP-choline, or anything else, to protect your brain, is *before* the damage occurs.

A Mitochondrial Program

The wide biochemical individuality of human beings makes it impossible to design a mitochondrial supplement program to suit everyone. The best we can do is study the amounts of nutrients used in controlled trials, amounts that protect the mitochondria without side-effects or known toxicity. Using these amounts as a base, we have developed the ranges in the table below for each nutrient. We have found these ranges effective in improving memory and movement, balance and reaction speed, in healthy individuals and in athletes.

In our **Brain Program** we tailor the amount of each nutrient to each person based on extensive individual analyses. I have no access to you the reader, so, any use you make of the table or any other information herein is at your own choice and sole risk. The best I can offer is access to the scientific references that can help you make an informed decision.

Table 5.2. Daily Supplement Ranges Used for Mitochondrial Protection by the Colgan Institute

Supplement	Dosage
R+ lipoic acid	200 – 800 mg
Acetyl-l-carnitine*†	500 – 2500 mg
N-acetyl-cysteine	200 – 400 mg
Idebenone	200 – 400 mg
Selegiline*†*	1.0 – 6.0 mg
CDP-choline	500 – 1000 mg

Taken in divided doses, half in a.m., half at noon, with food.
*† We do not take acetyl-L-carnitine or selegiline after 3 pm, because they stimulate the function of "get-up-and-go" neurotransmitters, dopamine and acetylcholine.
* Selegiline Use: We individualize selegiline by numerous criteria, but the most important are Biological Age and sex. See table 5.1 earlier in this chapter.

George Lucas mingled ancient legend and modern physics with artistic abandon to portray the Force in Star Wars. Nevertheless, the light sabers of the Jedi knights provide an elegant metaphor for the enormous power of the energy of the universe. The mitochondrion is not evolved enough to handle all this energy as it is released from food. So it damages the brain. New science is giving us powerful tools to better use the light.

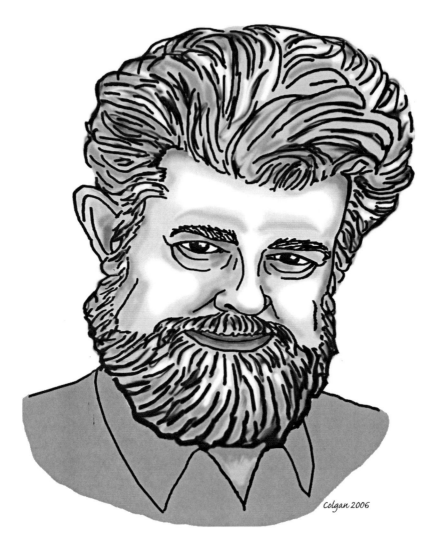

Colgan 2006

"May the Force be with you."

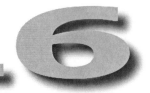

Nitric Oxide

Nitric oxide is one of the many gaseous chemicals in the human body which attest to the old jibe that we are full of hot air. It is manufactured by an enzyme called **nitric oxide synthase**. This enzyme turns the amino acid L-arginine into citrulline and nitric oxide, both of which serve multiple bodily functions. Throughout the brain, nitric oxide is an essential chemical messenger, improving communication between neurons, stimulating release of neurotransmitters, and promoting transmission and storage of information.[1,2]

Nitric oxide is also a free radical, what is called a **reactive nitrogen species (RNS)**, but it is relatively benign.[1,3] Like many other biochemicals, however, it can multiply out of control. Then it cooks your brain. It happens like this. Various stressors, such as banging your head against a brick wall, cause certain defensive genes to turn on, and the brain begins to manufacture pro-inflammatory gremlins called **cytokines**. These nasty little beggars stimulate billions of structures called glial cells, to produce large amounts of

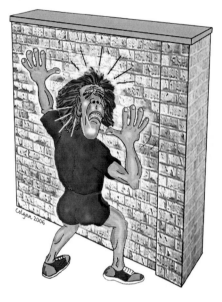

Banging your head, even very carefully, against a brick wall, induces formation of enough nitric oxide in brain cells to permanently damage your brain.

a particular form of nitric oxide synthase. It is termed inducible nitric oxide synthase, because it is induced by stress. This enzyme then gobbles up all the spare L-arginine and produces a ton of nitric oxide, which overwhelms other control chemicals and causes raging inflammation. Result, damaged brain cells all around.

If you bang your head ve-r-r-r-y carefully against a brick wall for years on end, as some martial artists do, then, after a while, the defensive genes continue to sleep through it, and no inflammation occurs. So you can take severe blows to the head without much damage. At least that's the theory. Don't try this at home.

By Thought Alone

You don't need a wall or any other blunt object to cause brain damage. A typical brain stressor common to modern urban life, is the automatic fear and anger reaction at a near miss on the freeway. The wise realize they are unhurt, calm down immediately, and move back to the real purpose of life, a state of joyful ease. Those who let their emotions balloon into "road rage," however, irreversibly damage their own brains.

Numerous animal studies show that fearful and angry thoughts readily cause brain damage, by the same process that occurs with the physical damage from banging your head on a wall. In a new study, representative of the evidence, De Cristobal and colleagues at Universidad Complutense, Madrid, restrained rats, but did not physically harm them. The rats went ballistic with fear and rage, and severely damaged their brains by huge production of inducible nitric oxide.[4]

Being rats, they could not understand what was going on, only that their lives appeared to be threatened. Being not quite as tied to present stimuli as rats, we can work out that fear and anger do not exist in any object or situation, but are creations of our own consciousness. Thus, in any event where no physical harm occurs, we always have the choice to avoid negative emotions. By now I hope I have convinced you, that by lifestyle choice alone, even your choice of thoughts, you can profoundly influence gene expression and either protect or endanger the physical structure of your brain.

Physical Damage

Air pollution provides a good example of a physical brain stressor just as damaging as a brick wall, yet unfelt and invisible. It is also impossible to avoid in urban life. In a typical recent study by the Toxicology Department of the University of North Carolina, researchers measured the brains of new-born dogs exposed to the air pollution of Mexico City, (worse than Los Angeles) and compared them with dogs living in an unpolluted area. The dogs breathing the polluted city air, showed large increases in the enzyme nitric oxide synthase, with a consequent cascade of inflammatory events that damaged neurons throughout their brains. They also showed deposition of plaque and neurofibrillary tangles, and increased apoptosis (cell death), very like the degenerative changes of the human brain found in Alzheimer's disease.[5]

Lillian Calderon and James Swenberg at the University of North Carolina, recently conducted follow-up studies on autopsied human brains from Mexico. Results showed that the people who had lived in cities with highly polluted air, had the same pattern of brain damage as the dogs.[6] These degenerative changes are classic signs of early Alzheimer's.

This evidence is recent and not yet extensive, but I venture to predict

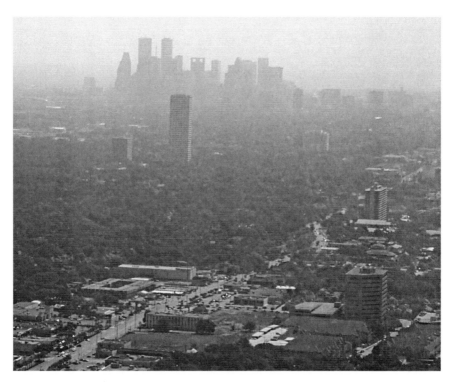

Figure 6.1. Air pollution damages your brain.
On a cloudless day in Houston, Texas...

that highly polluted cities, such as Los Angeles, New York, Chicago, Vancouver or Toronto, produce similar brain damage in everyone who lives there. I have urged readers in previous books to arrange their lives so as to flee the city, to protect their health, especially their children's health, against cancer and cardiovascular disease. These new discoveries of air pollution as an unavoidable urban source of brain damage, give you even more reason for treating cities as a nice place to visit, but you wouldn't want to live there.

The Glutamate – NO Link

As we saw in Chapter 3, fear, anger, and air pollution also damage the mitochondria and reduce the supply of ATP.[2,4,5] The protective electric fences around outer cell membranes lose power, and unwanted substances leak into the cell. Particularly opportunistic is the neurotransmitter glutamate, responsible for fast, excitatory neural transmission, just the sort of brain activity that increases in fear and anger situations. Glutamate attacks what is called the n-methyl-d-aspartate (NMDA) receptors on neurons, making a sort of hole through which calcium and other nasties can leak into the cell.[2]

Calcium is very nasty when it gets into the wrong place, as anyone who has had a heel spur or calcified artery can attest. In brain cells it converts an enzyme called **xanthine dehydrogenase** to **xanthine oxidase**, a process which produces a mass of superoxide free radicals.[7,8] Then all hell breaks loose as the excess nitric oxide, already being produced by the brain stressor, combines with the superoxide to make the extremely damaging free radical **peroxynitrite (0N00-)**. Peroxynitrite damages mitochondria, DNA, other proteins in brain cells, and any other tissues that get in its way.[7-9]

Some of these findings come from recent research on the brain damage caused by drugs such as methamphetamine, damage that is very like early Alzheimer's. In a representative study, Imam and colleagues at the US National Center for Toxicological Research, in

Jefferson, Arkansas, showed that peroxynitrite is the major culprit.[9] With every step of evidence, science is tying the brain damage caused by a wide variety of stressors to the major forms of dementia.

Links To Alzheimer's

Cholinergic neurons in the hippocampus of our basal forebrain, shown in Figure 6.2, express the neurotransmitter **acetylcholine**. These cells are more primitive in evolution than cholinergic cells in the cerebral cortex. They evolved in the brains of short-lived, ferocious animals and are designed for shorter, more violent life than those in the cerebral cortex. They have higher levels of nitric oxide to speed neural transmission for violent action, and lower levels of endogenous antioxidants because they did not have to last very long. So they are more vulnerable to damage and are the first to go in neurodegeneration.

It is exactly these hippocampul structures that show the most damage in Alzheimer's disease, with large numbers of dead and dying cells, amyloid plaque blocking neural transmission, damage to mitochondrial DNA, and useless tangles of neurofibrils.[10] In cell culture studies, the amyloid plaque itself causes further release of nitric oxide, thereby creating a vicious and progressive cycle of damage.[11] Alzheimer's patients also have increased brain levels of inflammatory cytokines, which as we saw above, increase production of nitric oxide even further.[12]

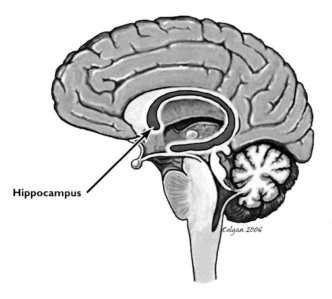

Figure 6.2. Mid-sagittal section of brain
with hippocampus superimposed.

Links To Other Dementias

Similar mechanisms have now been found in multiple sclerosis. Inflammatory cytokines stimulate glial cells to produce nitric oxide by way of the enzyme nitric oxide synthase, which then increases peroxynitrite to cause extensive mitochondrial damage.[13] Bagastra and colleagues at Thomas Jefferson University, recently found excess levels of nitric oxide synthase in every one of the brains of deceased multiple sclerosis patients, but in *none* of the control brains of people who had died without brain disease.[14] Induced Parkinson's disease in animals, in which the substantia nigra cells are deliberately damaged, shows the same pattern of enzyme activation.[15] So does Huntington's disease.[16]

Stroke patients also show large increases in inflammatory cytokines and nitric oxide synthase, even up to three months after the stroke.[17] Cerebral ischemia (restriction of blood supply) is also related to excessive glutamate stimulation of the NMDA receptor, with elevation of intracellular calcium and induction of nitric oxide synthase, which then raises nitric oxide levels.[8]

There are now hundreds of similar studies in the medical literature. In a major review of the research in October 2000, renowned expert on brain chemistry, Vittorio Calabrese, of the University of Catana in Italy, shows how this process occurs repeatedly with the stresses of usual urban life. He also reviews numerous other studies, showing that damage caused by excess nitric oxide is crucially involved in Alzheimer's, Parkinson's, Lou Gehrig's disease (amyotrophic lateral sclerosis, ALS) Huntington's disease, and multiple sclerosis.[1] Other researchers have shown that the same process of damage is a major determinant of the dementia caused by stroke and other forms of oxygen deprivation of the brain, and of various forms of brain seizure.[16, 17] Finally, the same process is implicated in common forms of epilepsy.[18]

Overall, the evidence shows that the brain degeneration caused in almost every one of us by excess nitric oxide, is also a major part of all common dementias, stroke, and even epilepsy. I have covered only a fraction of these new discoveries in this short chapter, but I hope it is a representative and convincing fraction. If you fail to protect the brain from excess nitric oxide, then all other efforts to maintain your intelligence will come to naught.

Protecting Yourself from NO

In commercial science, the reaction to the NO research is quite the opposite. Nitric oxide has numerous important functions in the human body from heart regulation to penile erection. When the latter became public knowledge in the late 1990s, athletes, especially bodybuilders, jumped at the chance to become more virile and more muscular by taking nitric oxide in a pill. A basic, profit-driven misapplication of biochemistry, these pills and potions have no lasting or healthy effect on muscle building, muscle recovery, or endurance. Even if they did, you should not load your body with nitric oxide if you want to keep your brain.

In real science, the discovery that excess nitric oxide is a major cause of the brain damage of usual aging, and of most major neurodegenerative diseases, has pharmaceutical companies scrabbling like rats up a curtain to be first to market with drugs that *inhibit* nitric oxide synthase, the enzyme that makes nitric oxide in your body. To formulate these drugs and to prove that they work, researchers give animals poisons that damage their brains in similar ways to the damage found in Alzheimer's, Parkinson's, and other diseases. Not my cup of tea, but that is the current method.

One particular toxin that produces Parkinson's-like brain damage in the substantia nigra, and the same symptoms, is methyl-phenyl-

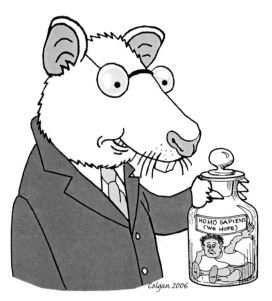

"Extraordinary creature."

tetrahydropyradine (MPTP). This poison works in two major ways. First, it increases nitric oxide production. Second, it reduces ATP production by the mitochondria, thereby reducing power to the electric fences protecting brain cells and their receptors. The fast, excitatory neurotransmitter glutamate we discussed earlier, then attacks the NMDA receptor, allowing calcium to leak into the cell and produce the superoxide free radical. Superoxide then combines with nitric oxide to make the free radical peroxynitrite. This Satan of free radicals promptly kills large numbers of cells in the substantia nigra, causing irreversible tremor, weakness, loss of balance, loss of muscle, and eventually dementia.

From numerous animal studies over the last five years, we know that anything which inhibits nitric oxide synthase can stop this whole scenario of damage. In a typical study, baboons were pre-treated with the nitric oxide synthase inhibitor **7-nitroindazole**. When subsequently given the poison MPTP, they were completely protected against cell death in the substantia nigra and showed no physical symptoms of Parkinson's.[19]

The man-made chemical 7-nitroindazole is not yet commercially available as a supplement and also has some nasty side-effects. But simpler, non-toxic substances work equally well. **Genistein**, extracted from soybeans (Figure 6.3), specifically inhibits nitric oxide production.[20] Genistein is also neuroprotective in mouse models of Lou Gehrig's disease (amyotrophic lateral sclerosis), and stroke, and in protecting post-menopausal women from Alzhiemer's.[21, 22]

Another inexpensive, non-toxic chemical that strongly inhibits nitric oxide synthase is **allicin**, extracted from garlic. In the latest study, Schwartz and colleagues at Tel Aviv Sourasky Medical Center in Israel, showed that allicin also inhibits the transport of arginine, from which nitric oxide is manufactured. So this simple herbal offers double-whammy brain protection.[23]

A third non-toxic herbal that regulates nitric oxide levels is **gingko**. In animal experiments, gingko effectively prevents the changes in nitric oxide levels caused by induced brain trauma, such as subarachnoid hemorrhage.[24] In studies of Alzheimer's patients, gingko stabilizes and, in less severe cases, improves cognitive performance.[25]

The final herbal I want to include in this chapter is the known liver protective agent **silymarin**. It does not inhibit nitric oxide production, but can indirectly stop nitric oxide turning into peroxynitrite. Silymarin specifically inhibits production of the enzyme **xanthine oxidase** which, as a side-effect, produces the superoxide radical, the other half of peroxynitrite.[26]

One of the so-called smart drugs, **aminoguanidine**, is also an inhibitor of nitric oxide synthase. This chemical has low toxicity and

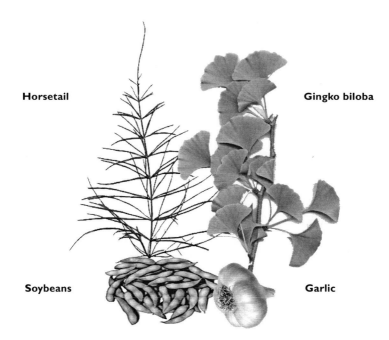

Figure 6.3. Genistein from soybeans, allicin from garlic, gingko extract and silymarin from horsetail, all inhibit excess nitric oxide production in the brain.

is now being tried against multiple sclerosis. In the mouse model of multiple sclerosis called encephalomyelitis, aminoguanidine suppresses nitric oxide production very effectively and reduces the disease.[27]

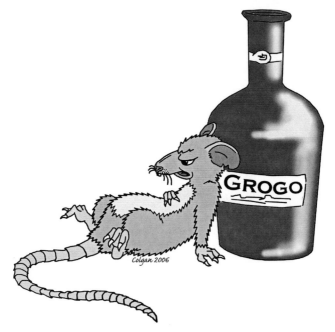

"Give me asprin or give me death."

Then there is **aspirin**. For the last 18 years most clients of the Colgan Institute over age 35, have been taking a baby aspirin each day to inhibit platelet aggregation and clot formation, and prevent heart attacks. Little did they know that they were also protecting their brains. Recent animal studies show that small amounts of aspirin, the equivalent in humans of one adult aspirin per day (325 mg), effectively prevent the rise in nitric oxide which occurs in response to fear and anger caused by stressors such as immobilization.[4]

Another non-toxic substance that inhibits the excess nitric oxide scenario is the omega-3 fat, **docosohexaenoic acid** in fish oil that we discussed in Chapter 5. This nutrient works by inhibiting release of inflammatory cytokines that trigger nitric oxide production by brain glial cells.[28]

The final protective item is the antioxidant **phenyl-butyl-nitrone (PBN)**, which acts at the inner membrane of the mitochondria, where energy is produced and has multiple protective roles.[29] Here we are concerned with inhibiting the damage caused by excess nitric acid. Robert Floyd and colleagues at the University of Oklahoma, have studied PBN and similar substances for the past 20 years. Their latest findings show that PBN effectively suppresses excess nitric oxide, both specifically by regulating inflammatory cytokines and generally by reducing brain inflammation.[30]

Thus we have an arsenal of substances with virtually no toxicity which can stop nitric oxide running amok in the brain, genistein, allicin, gingko, silymarin, aminoguanidine, aspirin, docosohexaenoic acid, and phenyl-butyl-nitrone. Unfortunately PBN is still not available commercially in effective supplement form. The range of each of the others that we use is shown in Table 6.1 below.

Table 6.1. Colgan Institute Program To Inhibit
Excess Nitric Oxide Production

Substance	Range of Daily Intake
Genestein*	10 – 50 mg
Allicin*	50 – 150 mg
Gingko*	200 – 500 mg
Silymarin*	150 – 450 mg
Aminoguanidine	150 – 300 mg
Aspirin	150 – 650 mg
Docosohexaenoic acid †	500 – 1000 mg
Phenyl-butyl nitrone (PBN)	Not yet commercially available in effective supplement form

* Extractions are not given for some herbals because of wide variations in chemistry of commercial products.

† This amount is in addition to the DHA in Table 10.1.

You need to add to these supplements by fleeing the city and its stressors. You also need to program your mind, as taught in the Quiet Mind program at the Colgan Institute, and outlined in Chapter 11 ahead, to eliminate negative emotions. Follow these steps, plus the strategies in previous chapters, and your brain will likely be good for more than a hundred years.

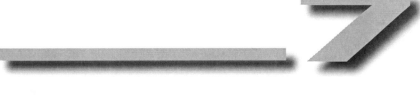

The Brain in Flames

Whack your neighbor on the nose, and it immediately glows red as arterial blood rushes to the area to enhance the supply of oxygen and nutrients. Whack it hard enough, and the offended proboscis swells like an onion as troops of the immune system pour in to mop up and remove dead and dying cells. As medieval medicine men used to say, the organ is "in flames."

Inflammation, as it came to be called, is an essential short-term process by which the body deals with all sorts of injuries, infections, and toxins, first by increased circulation of oxygen and nutrients, then by the inflammatory cascade of immune defense. In healthy people, once the repair and maintenance work is done, the tissues return to normal. With the usual aging syndrome that affects over 80% of Americans and Canadians, the inflammation lingers. It accumulates gradually and insidiously until it hampers normal

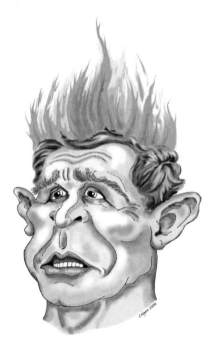

Brain "in flames"

function. As anyone who develops tennis elbow will tell you, this **chronic inflammation** can put a painful hitch in the whole game of life.

Chronic Inflammation

Most folk see chronic inflammation as inevitable creaks and twinges of age, and simply put up with it. Tolerance is an admirable quality, but in this case unwise. Recent discoveries show that chronic inflammation gradually destroys your joints, your organs, and especially your brain.[1]

Worse, the new evidence clearly shows that inflammation is a major cause of the leading degenerative diseases. The data are so strong that some scientists believe it to be *the* root cause. Now referred to as the CHAOS complex, chronic inflammation is known to underlie cerebrovascular disease (C), hypertension (H), adult-onset diabetes (A), osteoporosis (O), and stroke (S). Colon cancer and Alzheimer's disease have just been added to the CHAOS list.[1, 2]

We know now that all common brain diseases involve chronic inflammation. Alzheimer's got the nod simply because it is the most prevalent form. Unlike the rest of your body, the brain has no receptors for pain. So you don't feel a thing. Brain inflammation sneaks along silently, killing brain cells, destroying cognition, erasing memory. You don't even perceive it happening because the failing brain is the instrument you use to perceive. Perception slowly disintegrates.

No Fight or Flight

The ancient area of the hippocampus is especially vulnerable to inflammation. It evolved as a protective device in the first primitive mammals to enable them to recognize threatening situations and to react rapidly by fighting or fleeing.[2] Those animals survived whose hippocampus could react most quickly. They were our ancestors.

The fight/flight reaction, shown in Figure 7.1, is built into all of us. It occurs automatically by triggering the sympathetic branch of

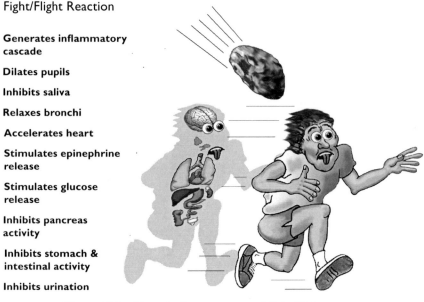

Fight/Flight Reaction

Generates inflammatory cascade

Dilates pupils

Inhibits saliva

Relaxes bronchi

Accelerates heart

Stimulates epinephrine release

Stimulates glucose release

Inhibits pancreas activity

Inhibits stomach & intestinal activity

Inhibits urination

Figure 7.1. Genetically programmed fight/flight response

the autonomic nervous system. The other half of the autonomic nervous system, the parasympathetic branch, is concerned more with rest and digestion. Sir Henry Dale received the Nobel Prize in 1936 for his discovery that these sympathetic nerves involved in fight or flight use acetylcholine as a neurotransmitter, as does your hippocampus.

This adaptive fight-flight reaction comes at high cost. The neurotransmitters and other chemicals that permit fast, excitatory reactions of neurons are at much higher levels in the hippocampus than in the cerebral cortex. Here we focus on three of the major chemicals involved. First is the excitatory neurotransmitter acetylcholine which, on its own, is not usually a problem. Second is the neurotransmitter glutamate, which promotes rapid excitatory activity. Third is nitric oxide, covered in Chapter 6, which improves the efficiency of neural transmission. Left on the biochemical boil, these three chemicals together inflame your hippocampus to the point of cooking.

Our culture imposes endless rules that forbid the fight or flight reaction programmed into your brain. It takes Zen mastery, or the Quiet Mind in Chapter 11, not to react with rage when someone rear-ends you, or Inland Revenue sends you a tax demand instead of the anticipated refund. But although the hippocampus is boiling, you have to sit and endure, unable to use up the accumulating brain chemicals in the violent action they were designed for. Thus we suffer repeated life situations, loosely called "stress," that generate vast numbers of inflammatory free radicals in the hippocampus and also induce genetic expression of inflammatory **cytokines**, plus excess nitric oxide, with no outlet for any of them.[3]

Top this off with inflammatory **zenobiotics**, toxins such as aluminum and mercury in the food chain and carbon monoxide and sulphur oxides in the air, and you have a potent witches brew for chronic hippocampul inflammation.[4] No wonder the US Centers for Disease Control report that Alzheimer's is the fastest growing category of disease over the last 20 years.[5]

Even at age 40, with most of your brain cells still intact, an inflamed brain doesn't work too well. Judgment becomes faulty, memory gets foggy, balance is off, and reaction speed declines. The good news is that new science, derived from old wisdom, offers great strategies to keep this inflammatory mechanism of brain damage under control.

Anti-Inflammatories Prevent Brain Inflammation

The universal remedy for the acute brain inflammation of a hangover is a couple of aspirin or ibuprofen, or other non-steroidal anti-inflammatory drugs (NSAIDs). Smart folk know that these drugs work a lot better if you take them *before* you start drinking. That is, they are a lot better at preventing inflammation than curing it.

NSAIDs work mainly by inhibiting the genetic expression of an enzyme called cyclooxygenase-2 (COX-2), which triggers the whole inflammatory cascade. Once the cascade is in full swing, as in a hangover, the NSAIDs no longer work very well except as a bit of an analgesic. This chemistry led scientists to think they might also work to inhibit the chronic brain inflammation of neurodegenerative disease.

The first evidence came from Patrick McGeer at the University of British Columbia. Together with Joe Rogers of Sun Health Research Center in Arizona, he sifted through a decade of hospital drug records. They found that arthritis patients who were regularly treated with strong anti-inflammatory drugs, were seven times less likely to develop Alzheimer's. Seven times![6]

These dramatic findings, albeit retrospective and uncontrolled, stimulated a rush of research. Rat studies quickly showed that simple aspirin given *before* the animals are subjected to psychological stress, such as restraint, inhibits three of the main mechanisms of chronic inflammation. Dissection of the rat brains showed that aspirin reduced the accumulation of nitric oxide and glutamate, and reduced the concentration of free radicals.[3]

Human Studies With Anti-inflammatories

Unlike rats, which are given no choice, people are somewhat reluctant to have their brains sliced and diced to show the anti-inflammatory benefits of drugs. Nevertheless, the indirect human evidence is compelling. A 15-year controlled analysis was published in 1997, using data from the Baltimore Longitudinal Study of Aging. This study has been running since 1958, measuring 2,300 people on a wide range of medical factors, including brain function, cognition, and memory. Walter Stewart and colleagues at Johns Hopkins University, and Jeffrey Metter at the US National Institute on Aging, examined the records of 1,686 subjects who were using anti-inflammatory drugs from 1980 to 1995. Their overall risk of Alzheimer's was *half* that of subjects not using the drugs. Ibuprofen (Advil) was the most used. Naproxyn sodium

(Naprosyn) was second.[6]

In 2001, a large prospective Dutch study, running for seven years, with 6,989 subjects, added further to these findings. The researchers showed that regular use of anti-inflammatories yielded a whopping 80% reduction in risk of developing Alzheimer's. The key finding is that the NSAIDs yield this benefit only if folk begin taking them regularly for years ***before*** they show symptoms of memory loss.[7] You don't have to take much, even one 200 mg ibuprofen a day shows the effect. But it has to get in there before the rot begins. As emphasized throughout this book, you have to get brain disease early – before it gets you.

Physicians are still reluctant to recommend daily use of NSAIDs to save the brain because of the side-effects on the gastrointestinal tract and kidneys. They recommend that the public wait for more studies. Wait? What a bizarre medical judgment. These drugs are routinely prescribed and shamelessly touted on television every day for any minor ache or snuffle. Yet they are hedged with dire warnings for the fatal disease of Alzheimer's — which doesn't wait for anyone.

Like everything else in this book, you use NSAIDs only at your own choice and risk. But folk on our brain program who do not have any contraindicating problem, such as gastric ulcers, have been using one 325 mg aspirin per day (or 200 mg of ibuprofen), taken with food, for the last 11 years without side-effects. I venture to predict that the awaited studies will show this strategy to be potent protection for the brain.

New COX-2 Inhibitors

In the 1990s there was a big race to market better COX-2 inhibitors than the existing NSAIDs. In 1999, two major pharmaceutical companies Merck and Pfizer introduced new arthritis drugs, **rofecoxib** (Vioxx), and **celecoxib** (Celebrex). There are several other "coxibs", but these two are representative. Hailed by the media as "safe aspirin," these drugs strongly inhibit inflammation without the gastrointestinal and other side-effects of NSAIDs.

Cyclooxygenase is a key player in the inflammatory cascade. It comes in two forms, cyclooxygenase-1 (COX-1) and cyclooxygenase-2 (COX-2). COX-1 is called the **constitutive form**, because it signals release of inflammatory chemicals as part of the body's normal immune reactions to toxins, bacteria, viruses, and injury. COX-1 is essential to your health. You do not want to inhibit COX-1.

Not discovered until 1992, COX-2 is called the **inducible form** of cyclooxygenase. It can be induced by all sorts of stresses and can continue at high levels long after the stress has ceased. To combat chronic brain inflammation, or any other inflammation, we aim to strongly inhibit COX-2, but leave COX-1 alone.

Unfortunately, we still don't know how to do it. All the NSAIDs, plus the new COX-2 inhibitors, also tend to whack COX-1 if you take too much of them. Therefore, they also whack your immunity and leave you at the mercy of every wandering microbe seeking an undefended lunch. That is exactly what happens to folk who overuse aspirin, ibuprofen, or naprosyn.[8]

Researchers did their best to design the new drugs to selectively inhibit COX-2 and leave immunity intact. The drugs worked well *in vitro* (in the test tube), but in living tissue they inhibit both COX-2 and COX-1, depending on the dose and the individual patient. The wide range of biochemical individuality between people makes correct dosage extremely difficult to determine.[8, 9] Too much and you inhibit the essential inflammatory cascade of immunity; too little and you have no effect.

Because of these fundamental problems of human chemistry, numerous people using the drugs for arthritis suffered terrible side-effects from rofecoxib and celecodib. Rofecoxib was withdrawn from the market in September 2004 after being found to increase the risk of heart attack and stroke.[10] In a big trial in 2004, researchers showed that 800mg per day of celecoxib increased the risk of cardiovascular trauma *three-fold*.[11] Celecoxib is now restricted, as are other forms of these drugs that are still on the market. They do not offer a solution for chronic brain inflammation.

Natural COX-2 Inhibitors

Inside the skull we have no idea of the right dose because chronic brain inflammation is symptomless and cannot yet be measured without dicing the brain. The coxibs were synthetic COX-2 inhibitors, man-made drugs. They never existed on Earth before. There is, therefore, no way your genome could develop mechanisms to deal with them. Consequently, they may bypass bodily defenses to create all sorts of mayhem.

What you really need is naturally occurring COX-2 inhibitors that were part of our environment when the human body evolved. Then it had the evolutionary time necessary to develop mechanisms to recognize them and control effects of overdose.

Are there such substances? Indeed there are. In all the hype about the coxibs, the media tend to forget that simple aspirin, the acetylated form of natural salicylic acid, is a COX-2 inhibitor originally derived from the bark of the white willow (*Salix alba*) (Figure 7.2). It was used by Aristotle over 2,000 years ago to ease pain and excess inflammation. Many other plants we commonly use as food also contain salicylic acid.

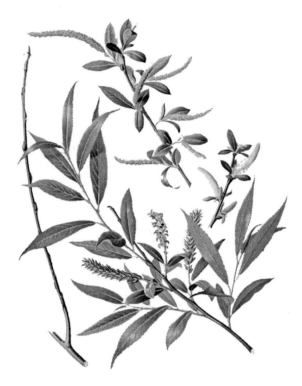

Figure 7.2. White willow (*Salix alba*). This deciduous tree contains large concentrations of salycilic acid in the bark. Aspirin was first synthesized from salycilic acid in 1860.

Pharmaceutical Profits

Why don't the pharmaceutical conglomerates simply make potent extracts from plants that contain COX-2 inhibitors? Because being natural substances, they cannot be patented under existing law. Without patent protection, there's little profit in selling them. Other companies can simply copy the formula and saturate the market.

To make their chop, drug companies need patent protection on their sales, so they can charge the typical mark-up of 20,000 to 50,000 times the cost of a pill. Otherwise, they could not afford their research facilities and thousands of employees. In contrast, companies that make herbal extracts typically have less than 20 staff, and the typical mark-up is five to ten times the cost of making the pill. In 2000 alone, the combined sales of just the two drugs, Vioxx and Celebrex, was **$5.7 billion USD**, yielding more profit than the combined sales of all herbals worldwide.[1]

I have touched on the politico-economics of drug development, not to deride the pharmaceutical giants, but rather to emphasize that scientists know a great deal more about natural chemistry than ever appears in the prescription drug marketplace. Though hailed by the media as a medical breakthrough akin to the polio vaccine, biochemists knew well from the start that the "coxibs" were only crude synthetic mimics of one action of natural chemicals. Nature operates with wider-ranging chemistry, using multiple mechanisms that enable plant COX-2 inhibitors to work a lot more safely than man-made drugs.

We were also exposed to these natural plant chemicals during our evolution, so our DNA has had the necessary time to develop mechanisms to deal with them. The salicylic acid of aspirin, for example, occurs widely in vegetables, though not in the concentration found in white willow bark. There are numerous other plant chemicals that inhibit COX-2 and NF Kappa B, plant chemicals that are widely distributed in edible plants and vegetables. We will focus on just a few of them, some of the aromatic plants that yield spice. These are complex substances concentrated in certain species found most abundantly in the Maluku Islands, formerly Moluccas, which lie near the Equator in what is now Indonesia, and other islands along India's Malabar coastline.

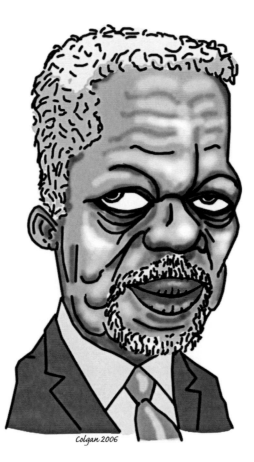

Colgan 2006

"Spice Islands? Never have trouble with
that lot. Must be something in them."

Secrets of Spices

Only now, in the 21st century, is science rediscovering secrets of aromatic spice plants that were known thousands of years ago. Ancient Greek, Roman, and Egyptian physicians had no idea of the chemistry, but they knew the effects. So potent were these plants, that merchant ships made arduous journeys to the Spice Islands and other distant shores, solely for cargoes of turmeric, cinnamon, ginger, cloves, and red pepper.

All these aromatics are strong anti-inflammatories. Extracts and inhalations were widely used internally and externally to soothe pain, inflammation, and mental disturbance. Throughout the arrogance of 19th and 20th-century medicine, which taught that its chemistry could design better drugs than Nature, much of this knowledge was discarded and lost. Today we realize that it is not so easy to meddle in the crucible of the Universe with our simian fingers. The new medicine of this century humbly acknowledges that **Nature made all the locks and holds all the keys**.

I am not talking herbal hocus-pocus here, the supposedly miraculous effects of plants that fill magazines and the internet but have never been scientifically validated. Only hard science can save your brain. Every conclusion I reach in this book is referenced to strong evidence from recent controlled studies in mainstream medical journals. I urge you to examine these listed references for yourself, to see whether I have made a good fist of it. You can view the abstracts on the internet. Simply enter "**entrez pubmed**" into any search engine, and – presto – you get free access to the US National Medical Library. Here we have only enough space to peek at a few representative findings.

The overriding control chemical in the inflammatory cascade is **nuclear factor kappa-B**, (**NF-kappa B** for short). This gremlin controls genetic expression of both COX-2 (inducible cyclooxegenase) and inducible nitric oxide synthase, the enzyme that causes overproduction of nitric oxide.[12] If we can safely control the action of NF-kappa B, then we kill two of the main inflammatory birds in the brain with one shot. Some delicious non-toxic plants can do just that.

At the Colgan Institute, we have followed and carefully analyzed the flurry of new research on spices because these plant extracts were traditionally used as anti-inflammatories, only to be discarded when patentable, man-made, profit-driven drugs appeared from about 1900 on. Spices have not yet been tested against chronic inflammation of the brain. But they have been tested in controlled trials against a wide variety of diseases: turmeric against colon cancer; cinnamon against diabetes, insulin resistance, and high cholesterol; gingerols against arthritic inflammation; cloves against diabetes; and red pepper (capsaicin) against arthritis. What binds these diverse diseases together is the excess production of COX-2 and NF-kappa B that brings chronic inflammation, pain and damage in all of them.

Turmeric Inhibits NF-kappa B

New science often comes from unexpected sources. One of these is a new experimental treatment of colon cancer. Colon cancer grows from the same out-of-control inflammatory processes that damage the human brain.[12, 13] Recent research shows that some herbal COX-2 inhibitors not only inhibit the growth of colon cancer, but can ***reverse*** and ***even cure*** the disease.[12-14] The strongest evidence is for chemicals contained in the pungent yellow spice turmeric.[14, 15]

But the turmeric you might have in your kitchen probably will not work. There are many varieties of turmeric, and only a few have proved to be strong inhibitors of NF-kappa B. Three extracts shown to be effective are **curcumin** from *Curcuma longa l,*[12, 13] **xanthorrizol** from *Curcuma xanthorrhiza Roxh,*[16] and **beta-turmerone** from *Curcuma zedoaria Roscoe.*[16] You need to use the exact extracts proven to work in controlled studies because, as with all science, God dwells in the minutest details.

It's not quite that easy. Turmeric works very well ***in vitro***, but as an oral extract for live humans absorption is negligible. To overcome the absorbtion problem, we use all three extracts combined with **piperine**. Piperine is extracted from peppercorns, the fruit of the pepper vine (*Piper nigrum*) (Figure 7.4). Daily dosage is hard to specify because herbals are poorly regulated and vary in potency between products. The best available is an 8% extraction from the rhizome. From the research, we estimate that a daily dose of

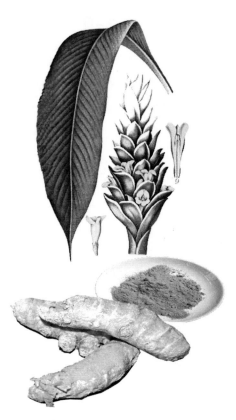

Figure 7.3. Turmeric. This pungent yellow spice
is a strong, non-toxic anti-inflammatory.

150 mg of each turmeric extract combined together with 50mg
of piperine might be effective. In any sensible amounts, turmeric
and its extracts show no evidence of toxicity. If you grind your
peppercorns at home and like pepper on your food, that is an
excellent way to get the piperine.

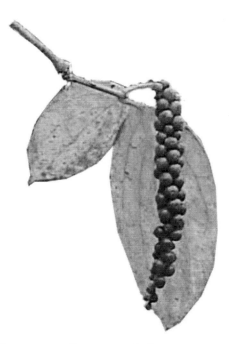

Figure 7.4. Pepper vine (*Piper nigrum*). Peppercorns are the source of piperine which aids absorption of plant anti-inflammatories.

Cinnamon Combats Brain Inflammation

A small pungent evergreen tree yields **cinnamon sticks** (*Cinnamomum verum*) from its bark (Figure 7.5). They are strong inhibitors of COX-2. The cinnamon you have in your kitchen or see at the supermarket probably will not work because it isn't real cinnamon. Most cinnamon sticks sold in stores are another much cheaper plant, called **cassia** (*Cinnamomum aromaticum*). The sticks look and smell similar, but cassia doesn't work as an anti-inflammatory.

You can test your cinnamon sticks easily. If you put a real cinnamon stick in a coffee grinder it will grind to fine powder right away. Cassia cinnamon sticks are much more fibrous and will not powder, but simply jam your grinder. A low-tech test but accurate.

The best new research on cinnamon comes from the US Human Nutrition Research Center in Beltsville, Maryland. In 2002 renowned scientist Richard Anderson and colleagues began

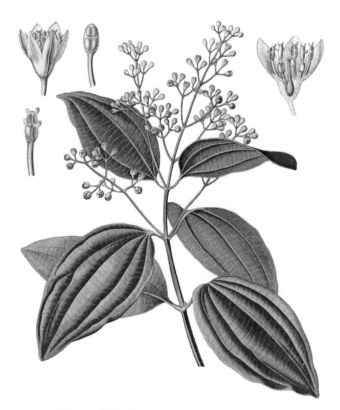

Figure 7.5. True cinnamon (*Cinnamomum verum*) is a potent anti-inflammatory.

examining effects of cinnamon on blood glucose, cholesterol, and triglycerides in 30 men and 30 women with adult-onset diabetes. They found that doses of 1.0 grams, 3.0 grams or 6.0 grams of cinnamon per day, dramatically reduced serum glucose, triglycerides, and LDL cholesterol (the clotter).[17]

By April 2006, the strong anti-inflammatory of cinnamon were confirmed by chemical analysis in two new studies reported at the Experimental Biology Conference in San Francisco, one led by Heping Cao of the Beltsville Human Nutrition Research Center and the other led by Stephanie Lampke of the University of California, Santa Barbara. We now know from the chemical structure and interactions of cinnamon, that it provides a definite aid in our bid to prevent inflammation of the brain.[18, 19] Dr. Anderson is getting studies underway to see its effects in inhibiting Alzheimer's.

How much cinnamon? First, you have to know that the processed cinnamon powder sold in jars as a herb is insoluble in water and probably will not work. Powdering real cinnamon will work a bit better. The easiest is to take the cinnamon in a capsule. We use 1.0–3.0 grams per day depending on the individual case. Three grams is about a teaspoonful.

Ginger Is Anti-inflammatory

Ginger (*Zingiber officianalis*) is a perennial plant often used as ornamental. Figure 7.6 shows the medicinal bit, commonly called ginger root, but actually an underground stem of the plant. Widely and effectively used to inhibit motion sickness, nausea, and vomiting, new research shows that 6-gingerol extract is also a potent anti-inflammatory.

As with cinnamon, the new research on this ancient herb didn't get going until this century. Earlier in the 1990s, studies on ginger with arthritis patients were generally a failure. I thought then that it was the wrong disease model to test this herb. We needed to see studies on insulin and lipid metabolism in which the inflammatory markers are much closer to what happens in the chronic brain

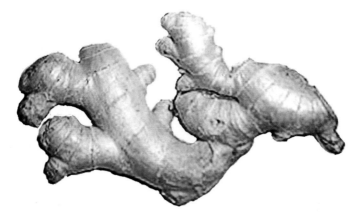

Figure 7.6. Ginger (*Zingiber officinalis*). The underground stem, popularly called "ginger root" provides 6-gingerol, a unique non-toxic anti-inflammatory chemical which protects the brain.

inflammation of aging. We picked up the first good hint in 2000. Bianca Fuhrman and colleagues at the Rappaport Institute in Haifa, Israel, showed that gingerol reduced LDL cholesterol levels and LDL oxidation by over 50%. That's big.[20]

By 2005 there were numerous reviews, including some research we had missed showing that gingerol is a good COX-1 and COX-2 inhibitor. For equivalently matched doses, it is better than aspirin because it has no adverse gastrointestinal effects. It also works by a different additional mechanism. We now know that gingerol inhibits the expression of the genes that activate inflammatory cytokines as well as those that activate inducible cyclooxygenase (COX-2).[21]

There are no standardized gingerol medicinals yet. You can, however, buy 5% extraction gingerol from Oriental suppliers. There are also no standard doses. With little to no toxicity, ginger, like other spices, is on the Food and Drug Administration GRAS list, (generally recognized as safe), so that is not a worry. From amounts used many studies we have zeroed in on a dose rage of 2.0–4.0 grams of ground fresh ginger rhizome or 400–800 mg of 5% 6-gingerol extract per day, as an additional and unique, naturally-occurring chemical that can protect the human brain.

Cloves Inhibit Inflammation

Some of the best cloves (*Syzgium aromaticum*) still come from Zanzibar in the Spice Islands. They are the dried, unopened buds of a small evergreen tree in the myrtle family, and shaped somewhat like old square-head nails. Shown in Figure 7.7, cloves contain the essential oil **eugenol**, which has been used traditionally and effectively in all sorts of remedies, especially for toothache. We became interested in eugenol because of recent research shows that it inhibits expression of the inflammatory cascade by blocking calcium channel transmission in dental nerves.[22]

Alam Khan at the Agricultural University in Peshawar, Pakistan, took the next step. In conjunction with Richard Anderson at the US Nutrition Research Center in Beltsville, he is studying the

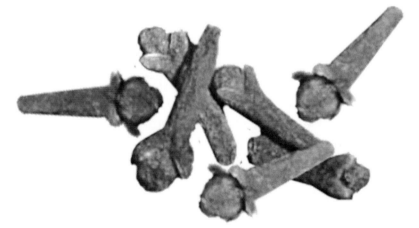

Figure 7.7. Cloves (*Syzgium aromaticum*) provide another unique anti-inflammatory for the brain, the essential oil eugenol.

effects of eugenol on insulin function in adult-onset diabetics. You will notice throughout this book that the fate of your brain, your insulin function, and your lipid function (and cardiovascular disease) are tied together by the state of your inflammatory cascade. In 2006 Dr. Kahn reported that patients treated with 1.0-3.0 grams of cloves per day, significantly reduced their serum glucose, their serum triglycerides, and their serum cholesterol in 30 days.[23]

The chemical mechanisms remain to be properly defined, but we are pretty confident that eugenol will prove yet another unique anti-inflammatory for the brain. No one knows what dose to use. From the evidence we have been able to piece together, 1.0-2.0 grams of cloves per day should provide a long-term effect. As they are GRAS foods, toxicity should not present a problem.

Capsaicin: Unique Anti-Inflammatory

The final spice that has some solid evidence to support its use is red pepper. The pungent oil of chili peppers is **capsaicin**. Used since ancient times for analgesia, the turn of the millennium brought a burst of new studies that now fill 500 research papers a year.

The usual bell peppers you see in the supermarket contain zero capsaicin. Capsaicin content is measured in parts per million which is then converted into what are called Scoville units. The hottest of the hot are habaneros with a score of 100,000–300,000. Far too hot for most people! Then come Scotch bonnets and Jamaican at

100,000–250,000 Scoville units. To understand how hot that is, cayenne pepper scores only 30,000–50,000. The heat experienced from capsaicin occurs because it stimulates pain and temperature receptors. Continued application to the skin causes long-lasting analgesia.

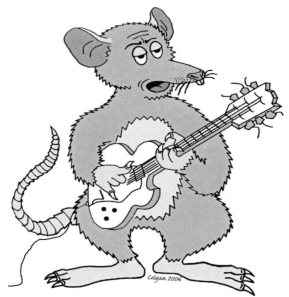

Red Hot Chilli Pepper

We became interested in capsaicin when research began to show complex and unique effects. To briefly summarize some highlights, there are four new developments. First, recent research has discovered a new neural receptor in the human system now called the "capsaicin receptor."[24] Second, from extensive studies the Food and Drug Administration has recently approved a capsaicin spray, which, when sprayed up the nose onto the nazal epithelium, relieves headaches that are resistant to NSAIDs. You can now buy various versions of this spray at your pharmacy. Third, research shows that capsaicin applied locally to the skin has anti-inflammatory effects at remote sites in the body. Fourth, capsaicsin affects one of the neuro-hormonal systems that regulates the hormone cascade.[25] We are pretty confident that capsaicin will prove a potent anti-inflammatory in the brain which uniquely inhibits inflammation pathways not accessed by other nutrients.

As with other spices, no one knows how much capsaicin to use long-term to help prevent chronic inflammation of the brain. From the huge pile of recent studies, it is only a minute amount. Pure capsaicin is extremely toxic and would burn a hole right through you. Even one drop in 100,000 dilution can raise blisters on the skin. We do not know of any commercial capsaicin remedy for use by mouth, but cayenne pepper is readily available, and you can add hot peppers to your diet. We use 250–500 mg of cayenne.

Docosahexaenoic Acid

The final brain anti-inflammatory I want to mention is the omega-3 fish oil, **docosahexaenoic acid** (**DHA**), that we have covered in earlier chapters. Completely non-toxic in any sensible amount, DHA is one of the essential fats that provide the long-chain fats that make up much of the structure of your brain. It's a real bonus to discover that it also protects the cells. Recent research shows that DHA has specific effects in inhibiting the production of the inflammatory cytokines that put the brain into a state of chronic inflammation.[26, 27] We use 500 - 1000 mg of it every day.

Table 7.1 shows a summary of our use of anti inflammatories that have documented effect in inhibiting excesses of the inflammatory cascade. As always, you make use of this information at your own choice and sole risk. The research is progressing rapidly, hopefully towards the day when apparently isolated fields of study finally focus on the most important instrument of health – the human brain.

Table 7.1. Colgan Institute Use of Anti-inflammatories

Substance	Range of Daily intake
Aspirin	325 – 650 mg
Turmeric	
Curcumin	150 – 300 mg
Xanthorrizol 8% extract	150 – 300 mg
Beta-tumerone 8% extract	150 – 300 mg
Piperine	250 – 50 mg
Cinnamon (powderd bark)	1.0 – 3.0 grams
Ginger (5% gingerol extract)	400 – 800 mg
Cloves (powderd)	1.0 – 2.0 grams
Cayenne (dilute capsaicin)	250 – 500 mg
Docosahexaenoic acid *	500 – 1000 mg

*This amount is in addition to the DHA specified in Chapter 6.

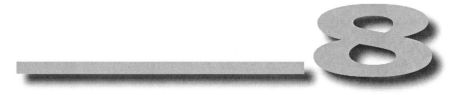

Parkinson's Puzzle

English physician James Parkinson first described the symptoms of Parkinson's in 1817.[1] He called it the "shaking palsy," but had no idea of its cause or how to treat it. It took another 150 years to solve the mystery.

In 1913, Friedrich Lewy discovered pink-staining, round globs in areas of dying nerve cells. Combined with physical symptoms, primarily resting tremor, loss of balance, rigidity, and slowness of movement, these **Lewy bodies** used to be a definitive diagnosis for Parkinson's disease. Today, some researchers consider them a separate phenomenon, the underlying factor in what is termed Lewy Body disease.[2] Some even consider Lewy bodies to underlie a whole group of different diseases. But these globs of damaged cells also occur in the brains of Alzheimer's patients, Parkinson's patients, in other dementias — and in some apparently healthy people. This increasing complexity of sub-categorization compromise is not a mark of great scholarship in the field.

The rest of Parkinson's has been split into grab-bag lots. There is idiopathic Parkinson's with, supposedly, no known cause. V-e-e-e-ry helpful. There *is* genetic Parkinson's, mostly related to an autosomal dominant gene which codes for a protein called alpha-synuclein.[3] Autosomal simply means that it occurs on a gene that does not determine sex. Dominant means that offspring have a 50% chance of inheriting it. This gene defect confers a tendency to develop Parkinson's in about 5–10% of cases. But only about half of those showing the genetic markers ever develop the disease. Also, the rate of Parkinson's in identical twins is no higher than among fraternal twins, so we are pretty sure that at least 90% of all cases are caused by life events or environmental trauma.[4]

There is also head-trauma Parkinson's, resulting from inflammation. The main gremlins involved are excess nitric oxide, over-expression of inflammatory cytokines, and decline of mitochondria.[5-7] We examined all of these factors and what to do about them as part of the brain damage of usual aging in Chapters 3–7. Finally, there is environmental Parkinson's, which we discussed in relation to pollution and neurotoxins that are factors in most brain diseases.

These multiple variants of Parkinson's have their advocates fighting over territory, symptomatology and, most of all, share of research funds. The result is we no longer have any definitive diagnosis for

Parkinson's.[8] The Michael J. Fox Foundation, which was founded in May 2000 by the celebrity sufferer of the disease and has funded some good research, announced in August 2006 that Parkinson's may not even be a disease at all![8]

Some folk are going to be annoyed with me for dismissing so much research in a single page. And indeed, it would take a whole book just to cover this one matter in detail. All else I can say here is that we have been watching this scene unfold for the last 30 years. It reminds me of the unworkable compromises of the Ptolemaic Universe, which, nevertheless, held sway for a thousand years. We tend to forget we are no smarter than all the medieval scholars who believed in it. Ptolemy's scheme fell immediately when subjected to the greater brain power and much simpler model of Galileo and Newton, which, in turn, fell immediately with the genius of Einstein.

I want to suggest an explanation of Parkinson's that better fits the science. The structural damage and the symptomatology of the disease are simply a part of the multiple-system brain damage of usual aging, damage that affects almost all of us. As I explained in Chapter 1, the symptoms of this brain damage that become dominant, and trigger a particular diagnosis, denote merely the structures most affected.

In the medical fog of geocentric compromises surrounding Parkinson's, however, the usual diagnosis follows the symptoms, and the treatment is almost always diagnosis-specific, symptomatic relief using the drug **levodopa (L-dopa)**. Unfortunately, unless you treat the whole brain, there is little hope of stopping or even slowing down its degeneration.

Substantia Nigra Damage

There is a smidgeon of logic behind levodopa. In 1919, a Russian neurologist, C. Tretiakoff, discovered that patients with symptoms of Parkinson's had lost dark-colored neurons in an area of the midbrain now called the **substantia nigra** (dark body), shown in

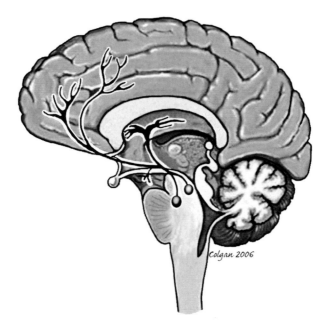

Figure 8.1. Mid-saggital section of brain showing substantia nigra and its projections to the midbrain and frontal cortex.

Figure 8.1. This area is part of the ancient mammal brain which mediates balance and control of voluntary movement. But it was not until the 1960s that researchers showed how Parkinson's symptoms, especially tremor and loss of balance, are caused by progressive death of nigral neurons which supply our brains with the essential neurotransmitter **dopamine**. Levodopa floods the brain with dopamine.

In a normal brain, Levodopa would produce a frenzy of overactivity. By the time a Parkinson's case has come to notice, however, there are not enough dopamine-producing cells left for the brain to over-react. The drug does help the remaining cells to function a bit longer, but does zero to prevent further cell death or slow the progress of the disease. Far too little, far too late.

Nigral neurons die off with age in almost every one of us. The most accurate predictor of Parkinson's, by far, is simply how long you have lived. Figure 8.2 shows that, between ages 55 and 65, the incidence triples. And by age 75, it increases almost nine-fold.[3] Parkinson's is simply part of the damage of the brain with age that would eventually get all of us, were we not to die of something else beforehand. Unless you treat the whole brain, you haven't got a hope.

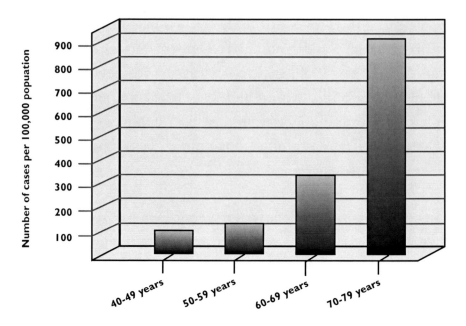

Figure 8.2. US incidence of Parkinson's. Incidence increases three-fold between ages 59 and 69 and almost nine-fold after age 70.

Rate of Loss of Nigral Cells

You have roughly 400,000 nigral neurons at birth, and that's about your lot for life. Only rarely do they divide or replicate. The average healthy brain loses up to 20,000 nigral cells per decade after age 25. So in 50 years, by age 75, you have lost up to 100,000 nigral cells, about 25% of your supply. By then you are getting shaky. Whether Parkinson's symptoms become apparent before we die of something else depends on the *rate* of nigral cell loss.

At first, the victim may notice only slight symptoms, such as hand tremor on picking up a cup of tea, and dismiss them as stress or fatigue. By then about 15–20% of the nigral neurons are already dead, and it is time to aggressively treat the disease. Otherwise, it progresses inexorably to shaking of the limbs, muscle wasting, loss of bone mass, loss of balance, rigidity and slowness of movement, difficulty in initiating voluntary movement, and finally loss of speech and movement altogether.

We know now that this silent, symptomless degeneration is happening to all of us. Parkinson's is diagnosed in over 1,000,000 people in the US alone. Prevalence of the disease is increasing rapidly throughout the Westernized world. It is always fatal, usually after a long illness.

Environmental Causes of Parkinson's

There is growing belief among researchers that the sudden increase in Parkinson's is caused by the man-made chemicals, drugs, and pesticides, collectively called **zenobiotics**, that now pervade our urban and suburban environments. Some people subjected to neurotoxins show rapid nigral cell loss and have *triple* the average risk of Parkinson's.[4] In these folk the disease begins to show by age 40 – 45.

Some of the best evidence that environmental toxins trigger Parkinson's is its uneven distribution. Even allowing for age and other confounding factors, prevalence (that is the number of people alive with Parkinson's in a population at any one time) varies widely state to state and province to province in North America. In Canada, for example, the overall prevalence of Parkinson's is close to one in about every 100 adults. But in British Columbia, prevalence is nearly 50% higher: one adult in144.[10] In the United States prevalence is much lower: one adult in about 250.[11]

What are the zenobiotics involved? We now have hard evidence against pesticides, herbicides, fungicides, and polychlorinated biphenyls (PCBs).

The latest large-scale controlled study of pesticide exposure and Parkinson's in the general public was released on 26 June 2006 by Alberto Ascherio and colleagues at Harvard's School of Public Health. They examined the medical records of 143,000 people. Their results confirm earlier reports that pesticide exposure is a major risk factor for the disease. After accounting for all other risk factors, those reporting exposure to pesticides, most often farmers, ranchers, or fishermen, but also including suburbanites, had a 70% increased risk of developing Parkinson's.[15]

The research on fungicide exposure took a leap in 1992 when small farming towns with heavy use of fungicides showed up to five times the national average prevalence of Parkinson's.[4] Since then, a flurry of research has shown nasty results. Strong evidence shows that commonly used fungicides freely sold for vineyards, vegetable farms, stock farms, suburban homes, golf courses, and public parks, preferentially target the substantia nigra and cause permanent irreversible damage to nigral cells.[12-14]

Because of the very widespread use of fungicides, like maneb for example, no individual knows just how much exposure they have had. Researchers call fungicides "silent toxicity" because, even after a number of exposures, there are no symptoms. There is a large nigral cell loss that shows on brain imaging, however, We also know that fungicides bioaccumulate, that is, they stay around and intensify their toxicity with re-exposure. Leading researchers now fear that the crop reaped from our careless use of fungicides is showing now, years after exposure, as a large increase in Parkinson's. The largest part of this effect on the public is yet to come. That's one big reason to begin to protect your nigral cells right now to slow the loss.

Poly-chlorinated biphenyls (PCBs) are also a problem. They were used freely in manufacture of electrical equipment from 1930-1980. When they started turning up in Antarctic penguins, folk began to get worried. PCBs are extremely persistent in the environment and cause all sorts of disease, but were not effectively banned until 1990. Even now, new "spillages," i.e., illegal dumping, of PCB waste occurs frequently n the US and Canada.

New research on PCB toxicity was reported from 2004-2006 by Lisa Opanashuk and colleagues at the University of Rochester School of Medicine in New York. The work shows that even small exposure (that's all of us) selectively reduces brain dopamine levels and causes nigral cell death.[16, 17] One more reason to begin now to protect your substantia nigra.

Environmental pollution will get a lot worse before it gets better. The solution we have discussed is two-fold: flee the cities and aggressively protect your brain. We have covered most of that protection in Chapters 5-7. It is summarized in Chapter 10.

Drink Coffee

There is one extra wrinkle. For about 20 years now, we have been collating reports that coffee inhibits Parkinson's. We were interested because the caffeine in coffee belongs to a chemical group called **xanthines**. One important xanthine in the human brain is adenosine, which we have discussed in relation to adenosine triphosphate, the energy molecule. Caffeine inhibits some adenosine receptors, causing dopamine levels to increase.

Until the last five years, the research was spotty. Now we have some good data. G. Webster Ross and colleagues at the University of Hawaii analysed the data from a 30-year follow-up of 8,000 Japanese Hawaiian men. Those who never drank coffee showed a massive five times the risk of developing Parkinson's.[18]

It doesn't affect only Japanese men. A large follow-up study by Alberto Ascherio and colleagues at Harvard analysed the records of 135,000 people of mixed ethnicity. They found that men who drank coffee regularly cut their risk of Parkinson's almost in half. The lowest risk occurred with moderate coffee intake of 1–3 cups per day (Figure 8.3). Beyond that level, risk rose again.[19] We are now confident that coffee is protective against Parkinson's.

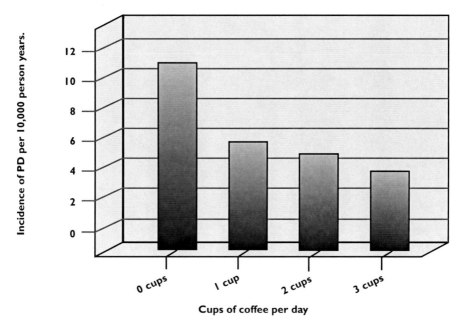

Figure 8.3. One to three cups of coffee per day reduces the risk of Parkinson's.

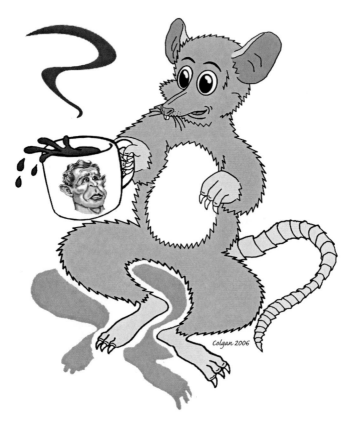

"Wow! Getting shaky."

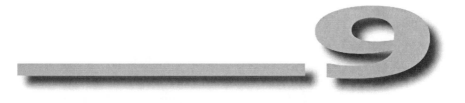

Alzheimer's Alert

O n the 10th of August, 1906, triumphantly puffing his constant cigar, German physician Alois Alzheimer announced his brilliant discovery of the disease that now bears his name. He presented the case of a woman, Frau August D., who died at age 51 with profound memory loss and organ failure. During treatment Dr. Alzheimer wrote,

> *Her behavior was dominated by total helplessness. She was confused as to time and place. At times she was delirious and carried parts of her bed around screaming for her husband and daughter.*

After death he dissected her brain and found the **neurofibrillary tangles** in the structure of nerve cells and the accumulation of **amyloid plaque** in the hippocampus that define Alzheimer's disease.[1, 2]

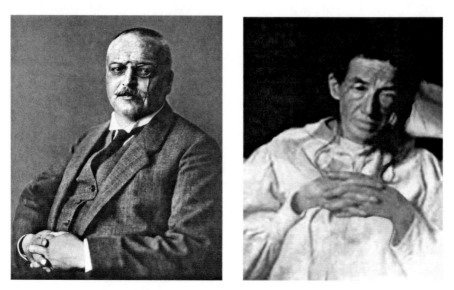

Figure 9.1. Dr. Aldous Alzheimer and his patient Frau August D, from whom he defined the disease that now bears his name

Little did Alzheimer suspect that he was describing damage we now know is present in some measure in the brains of ***almost all*** elderly folk. The only difference is that most folk usually die of other diseases before the brain damage becomes sufficiently advanced to be diagnosed as dementia.

Alzheimer's Strikes Almost Everyone

The Oregon Brain Aging Study is representative of a burgeoning pile of new evidence that the damage of Alzheimer's is happening to all of us. In somewhat macabre fashion, this very long-term research selects healthy, middle-aged volunteers who show no cognitive decline. Then they give these typical citizens comprehensive tests of memory and intellectual capacity, which are repeated on a regular basis until they decline and die. Mostly, they die of other disease, not dementia. At death their brains are removed and dissected. ***Every one of them*** shows neurofibrillary tangles and accumulation of amyloid plaque, especially in the ancient brain area of the hippocampus.[3, 4]

Most important, the degree of decline in memory and cognition in these people is directly correlated with the amounts of plaque and tangles in their dead brains.[3, 4] The evidence is now clear: the damage found in Alzheimer's disease is part of the brain damage of usual aging that will infect the mind of every person who fails to protect their brain.

The saddest and most controversial part of this book is what we are doing about it. Very little. In attempts to soften the blow and sweep the Alzheimer's epidemic under the carpet, medicine has come up with numerous names for early diagnoses of dementia that avoid the dreaded word "Alzheimer's." Common medical niceties are **age-associated memory impairment** (AAMI) and **mild cognitive impairment** (MCI). Such terms have less initial emotional impact on the patients and their families, but are disastrous in the long run. They encourage "watchful waiting" or perfunctory treatment with cholinesterase inhibitors such as donezepil. These drugs relieve some of the symptoms but do nothing to stop the disease. Yet most researchers realize well that the earliest evidence of an aging person "losing it," is *the* critical point when there is still a chance to save the brain. Instead, in many, many cases, the disease is left free to progress, as it inevitably does, until Alzheimer's symptoms become obvious.

From 32 years of studying brain function, we are firmly convinced that a large proportion of diagnoses of age-associated memory impairment, and similar terms, are really looking at early Alzheimer's, often with attendant Parkinson's disease as well. Immediate, intense treatment at that early stage is the only hope of preventing the patient sinking into dementia.

By now the informed reader will realize that I am in fundamental disagreement with the official government view of Alzheimer's. The most public voice for the disease, the American Alzheimer's Association, states unequivocally:

Alzheimer's disease is not a normal part of aging.[5]

The Canadian Alzheimer's Society and the US National Institutes of Health use exactly the same sentence in their explanations of Alzheimer's.[6,7] In fact, all three organizations seem to be quoting from the same notes. As long as this official view prevails, there will be no effective treatment. Meanwhile, the number of folk in America and Canada who are developing Alzheimer's is spiraling out of control.

Why do they ignore the last decade of research? The simple explanation is the patients they encounter and study. Their medical specialists never see the start of the disease. Their standard tests are scary. You have to be so far gone to fail them, it's all over. Every Joe Public who believes he still has his marbles keeps well away from them.

I have a great deal of respect for the caring work these organizations do with people who have been diagnosed with the disease. But those are the only people who come to their attention. They have little experience with people who have "just become a bit forgetful," or "now find the mall confusing," or "can't stand the traffic any more," or any one of the many similar epithets that cross my desk from family members. These reports are often years in advance of, finally and reluctantly, being forced by the progress of the brain degeneration of aging to attend a specialist for diagnosis.

I have no axe to grind here. I wish that the government view was correct and that most of us were not going to lose our brains to aging. The new science, however, is sobering. All that I ask is that you read the references given herein for yourself, so at least you get the scientific picture.

Astronomical Increase in Alzheimer's

Alzheimer's didn't even feature in the top twenty diseases in 1980. Since then it has jumped from nowhere to become the 8th leading cause of death in America, with a 23% jump in prevalence in 1999 and a 14% jump in 2000.[8] The Alzheimer's Association reports that one in every ten Americans now has a family member or relative with Alzheimer's.[5] Figure 9.2 shows the current prevalence and estimated rise in Alzheimer's in the US. This is one of the moderate estimates backed by the US government. Some researchers believe it should be much higher. Even taking the moderate figures, Alzheimer's is increasing faster than any other category of disease,

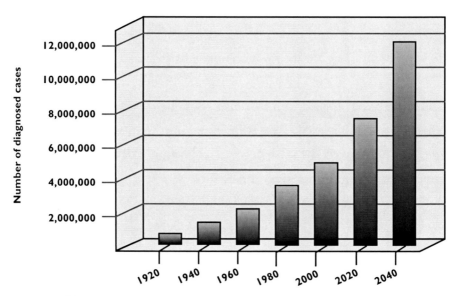

Figure 9.2. Prevalence of Alzheimer's disease and estimated increases in the number of diagnosed cases to 2040.[9]

and the rate of increase is accelerating.[9]   Unless there is a radical improvement in health policy, we can expect the number of cases to double in the next 20 years.   That will total over 10 million people with the disease.

Mindful of public panic, the US Centers for Disease Control have tried to explain part of the current increase as better diagnosis from 1998 on, but their own figures, graphed in Figure 9.2, show clearly the steep rise to epidemic proportions over the last 20 years.   If any other disease showed such a jump, such as AIDS, for example, which is minor in America by comparison, there would be dramatic public action sufficient to topple government.   But the saddest part of Alzheimer's is its victims don't have enough brains left to defend themselves.   Most relatives accept the medical advice that the fate of their loved ones is inevitable, which it is by the time they get bad enough to be diagnosed.

Remember, only about 10% of cases carry defective genes for the disease, and only half of those ever develop it.   It's hardly genetic. As the 2000 Report of the US National Institutes of Health states, most Alzheimer's cases are caused by cumulative brain damage that occurs during life.   And the biggest risk factor is age, that is, being around long enough for the accumulating damage to become sufficient to shatter your mind.[10]   As Western medicine and culture becomes more and more successful at keeping folk alive, a lot of us are now around a lot longer.

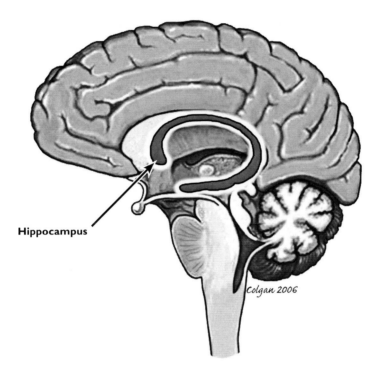

Hippocampus

Colgan 2006

Figure 9.3. Mid-saggital section of human brain showing the hippocampus. The hippocampus begins to show degeneration in almost everyone by about age 35.

For the more than 5,000,000 diagnosed cases of Alzheimer's in the US today, and the estimated 4,000,000 undiagnosed cases, plus the 500,000 estimated cases in Canada, about all that current medicine can offer is symptom relief and sympathy. Once this dread disease has you in its grip, treatment is mostly palliative, dementia and death inevitable. ***The time to stop Alzheimer's is as early as possible in adult life, when most of the cells in your hippocampus are still alive and kicking.***

Death Of The Hippocampus

The primary damage in Alzheimer's is loss of hippocampal cells that provide the essential neurotransmitter **acetylcholine**. It happens to almost all of us as we age. We know now that the average rate of loss of these cells in otherwise healthy people is about 4% per decade after age 25.[10] This loss is detectable as memory decline after one decade, that is, by age 35.

Some folk lose hippocampal cells at a faster rate. These are mostly among the 5% of Alzheimer's cases with a familial disposition. New studies using **magnetic resonance imaging** (MRI) of the brains of some cases who have genetic defects for Alzheimer's, have found massive hippocampal cell losses, up to 20% per decade.[11] These brains are in the throes of early Alzheimer's in one decade, by age 35 – 40. Severe hippocampel cell loss is shown in Figure 9.4.

When someone suspects Alzheimer's and asks for medical help, their physicians generally do not use brain imaging. Most of these folk are prescribed one of the drugs that inhibit an enzyme in the brain called **cholinesterase**. This enzyme breaks down the neurotransmitter acetylcholine. As we saw in earlier chapters, acetylcholine is emitted from the axons of the cells to pass information to the dendrites of other cells. It is *the* vital chemical for memory.

In normal young adult brains, the hippocampal cells make plentiful acetylcholine to support memory, and the normal job of

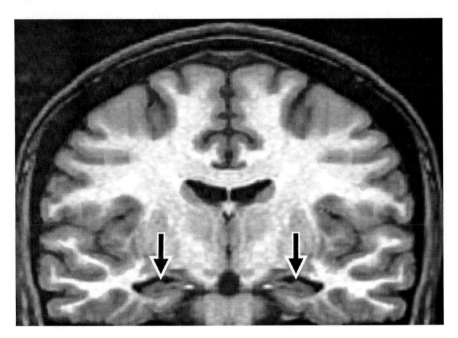

Figure 9.4. Brain imaging showing hippocampal atrophy (arrows).
Normal brains do not show empty "holes" around the hippocampus.

cholinesterase is to prevent the level of acetylcholine becoming too high. It does this job very well. When 30–40% of hippocampal cells have died, however, acetylcholine levels decline critically, and memory hardly functions any more.

So you can see how crude this drug treatment is. All it does is boost the level of acetylcholine. The dead cells don't revive. The dying cells continue to die at an ever increasing rate. The information flow from the remaining live cells gets through a bit better with the drugs, but that's it. This is the same treatment given to most older people diagnosed with Alzheimer's.

The problem is that cholinesterase inhibitors treat only one of at least six main mechanisms of brain damage in Alzheimer's, all the mechanisms of brain degeneration we have examined in earlier chapters. Current drugs reduce symptoms for a year or two, but do **nothing** to stop or even to slow the death of cells or the progress of the disease. After about five years of such treatment of folk with familial markers for Alzheimer's, magnetic resonance imagery of the brains shows that they have lost about another 20% of their hippocampal cells. By then, Alzheimer's has become obvious and irreversible, and treatment next to useless.[11-13]

Circling The Wagons

The common response to Alzheimer's in American society is denial. No one wants to know that a loved one who has become forgetful is on the verge of dementia. With the best of intentions, many families delay presenting a parent or relative for treatment as long as possible, often until more than 20% of the hippocampus is dead. By doing so, they unwittingly ensure that the disease is irreversible.[7-9] To stop Alzheimer's, you have to begin protecting the brain aggressively at the very first sign of memory loss, and preferably long before the first symptom.

You may be wondering what this sad scenario has to do with you, who have no familial disposition for Alzheimer's and are losing only about 4% of hippocampal cells per decade. Remember, even a 4% loss causes memory decline. In five decades, by the time most folk are 75 – 85, they have lost 20% of the hippocampus, and are in early Alzheimer's. And, long before that, their brains have stopped working well. To help you prevent this decline, we will review each major brain problem in Alzheimer's, and how we can intervene to prevent it. The good news is the new brain science is becoming adept at prevention.

Neurofibrillary Tangles

The first problem in Alzheimer's is aging damage to the cell structure. Inside each neuron there are many **neurofibrils**, tubular rods that form the structural skeleton of the cell. Neurofibrils also act as guides for transport of nutrients and neurotransmitters flowing from the cell body to its axon and dendrites. These neurofibril rods occur in parallel lines, formed like train tracks to guide the flow of chemicals. A protein called **tau** acts like railroad ties to hold the tracks apart and parallel.[6]

All well and good, except that the hippocampus in our brains evolved in short-lived, primitive mammals, as discussed in Chapter 2. In these creatures the hippocampus served to help them recognize threatening situations and either fight or run away. It is not designed for, nor robust enough, to withstand the stresses of our extended lifespan, especially the emotional restrictions imposed by our culture, and the man-made pollution we have spread throughout the Earth.

Culture and Pollution

Today we face repeated threatening situations such as rush-hour freeway driving, but can neither fight nor flee. We have to sit and endure, while our ancient mammal limbic system is biochemically boiling. We know now that many of these cultural norms cause hippocampal damage. The human brain was not designed to live in tightly packed cities.

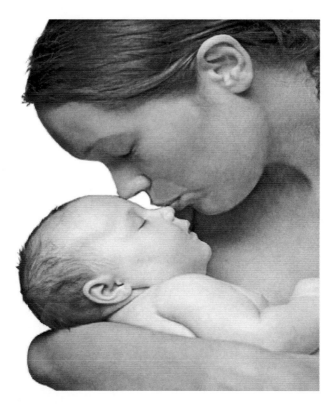

Figure 9.5. Breast milk in the US and Canada is so polluted it would be illegal to take it across a state line in any other container.

And, in any urban or suburban area, there is nowhere to run and nowhere to hide from pollution. The best marker is human breast milk. From 1990 to 2002, breast milk of mothers tested in the United States and Canada, was so polluted with man-made chemicals, that it would be illegal to transport it across a state line in any other container.[14, 15]

Under these stresses, especially from the DNA damage they cause, the brain produces a defective form of tau. Part of its genetic pattern is missing. This truncated tau cannot hold the myofibrils apart. Figure 9.6, taken with the newly developed laser scanning confocal microscope, allows us to see this brain damage with great clarity.[16] New fibrils grow twisted together, forming useless neurofibrillary tangles. Nutrients and neurotransmitters cease to flow, causing degeneration of the cell body and its axon, and eventual cell death.

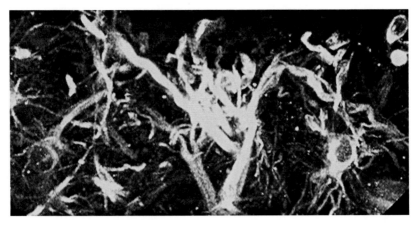

Figure 9.6. Neurofibrillary tangles in Alzheimer's disease.

From Mice To Men

Science confirmed the process of neurofibril damage in Alzheimer's only in the mid-1990's. Researchers bred genetically modified mice (Figure 9.7), whose DNA is altered to cause overproduction of the particular defective form of tau found in demented human brains. These mice develop neurofibrillary tangles and senile plaque in the hippocampus.

The mice also show damage in the substantia nigra and striatal areas, almost identical to that found in Parkinson's disease, including damage called **Lewy's bodies**, which, as we saw in the last chapter, is a defining characteristic of Parkinson's. New research has also found Lewy bodies in human Alzheimer's patients. These findings

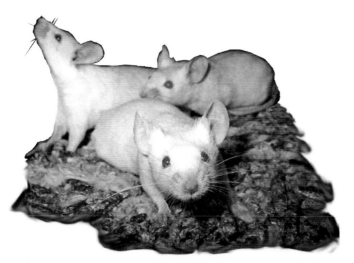

Figure 9.7. Transgenic mice, specially bred with defective DNA, begin to develop Alzheimer's-like changes in the brain shortly after birth.

are strong confirmation of the close relationship between the two diseases that I have stressed throughout this book.[17-19]

The transgenic mice are bred especially with defective DNA, so that their brains produce defective tau from birth. But normal human brains do not, at least in the first 25 years of life. So how does it occur in almost everyone? The answer that has gained strong research support over the last five years, is the focus of this book: **the DNA of normal brains is progressively damaged by free radicals.**

Amyloid Plaque

Tau is only one of several proteins that are abnormally produced in Alzheimer's.[6] Here we will examine only one of the others, the most important one, **beta-amyloid.**

Your brain produces what are called **amyloid precursor proteins**, which are essential for the repair of cell membranes. After about age 25, however, small fragments begin to break off these proteins inside the brain and accumulate as insoluble plaque in axons, and in the synapses between cells. This plaque, shown in Figure 9.8, impedes neural transmission, much like plaque in arteries impedes blood flow. When neural transmission ceases, the cell dies.

Amyloid plaque has a second damaging effect. In the normal brain, a continuous essential process called **apoptosis**, removes

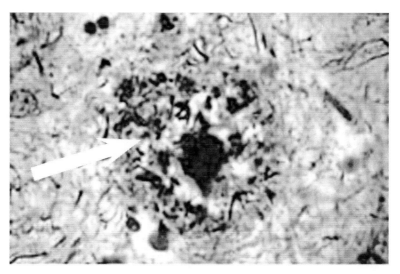

Figure 9.8. Amyloid plaque in a brain with Alxheimer's.

sick and dying cells by killing them off for removal by the immune system. Beta-amyloid causes genetic expression of an enzyme called **caspase-2** that causes apoptosis to go wild and kill healthy cells too. So, what is a normal scavenging process becomes predatory and literally eats your brain.[20]

The worst news about amyloid plaque is that it begins to accumulate, and sets these disease processes in motion, silently and without symptoms, long before there is measurable cognitive decline.[16] That is one big reason the Colgan Institute advocates beginning a brain program as early in adult life as possible. Most of us have been taught to protect our teeth from plaque, and do it every day. Yet we can easily replace or even do without teeth. You can't do without a functioning brain.

Protection From Plaque

The great news is we now know two precise mechanisms of degeneration by which amyloid plaque accumulates. The first is DNA damage. In Alzheimer's the accumulation of plaque is accelerated. In one familial form of the disease, the gene that encodes for amyloid precursor proteins is defective. Amyloid plaque accumulates from an early age, and Alzheimer's disease usually manifests by adulthood.

Children with Down's syndrome also show accelerated accumulation of amyloid. In these folk, dementia often occurs by age 40.[10, 21] It is likely that their genetic defect, which affects almost every system in their bodies, also causes production of defective amyloid precursor proteins.

These genetic defects occur in Alzheimer's and Down's syndrome on a continuum of severity. In some people, they produce such a quantity of defective amyloid precursor proteins that dementia and death occur in childhood. In others, the gene defect can be detected, but causes no apparent damage until mid-life or later.

A similar continuum of severity occurs in genetically "normal" brains. Some folk are subjected to such a free radical burden in early life, that the resulting DNA damage causes production of abnormal amyloid precursor proteins and cognitive decline by mid-life. Others suffer much less DNA damage, and beta-amyloid plaque does not impact cognition until their 70's or 80's, or later. So, our first task is to protect the gene which encodes for amyloid precursor proteins from damage by free radicals. We examined exactly how to do that in earlier chapters

The second degenerative mechanism by which amyloid plaque accumulates is the decline in glucose metabolism in the brain with usual aging. As we saw in Chapter 4, in almost everyone, production of adenosine triphosphate (ATP), our basic energy molecule, declines from about age 25 to about 50% of its optimum level by age 65 – 75.[22] Amyloid precursor proteins are normally incorporated into the brain cell membranes to help repair them. This incorporation is dependent on sufficient ATP being available.

As we get older and ATP declines, the whole brain is competing for amyloid precursor proteins. There is insufficient ATP to incorporate enough of these proteins into cell membranes to maintain normal brain structure. Studies at Basel University Medical School in Switzerland, show that they hang about unused until normal protein degradation processes breaks them into fragments. These fragments then accumulate as insoluble amyloid plaque.[23]

That's not all. Failure of the brain to incorporate amyloid precursor proteins into cell membranes causes degeneration of the membranes and eventual cell death. So, to prevent the accumulation of beta-amyloid and protect both the flow of neural transmission and the integrity of the cell membrane, our second task is to maintain ATP production throughout life. We covered our brain program to do that in Chapter 5.

Acetylcholine Decline

The major neurotransmitter driving information through the hippocampus is **acetylcholine**. As we have seen, it is critical for processing memory, especially short-term memory. As part of the brain damage of usual aging, the level of acetylcholine declines. This decline occurs by numerous mechanisms, from loss of hippocampal cells to loss of ability of the remaining cells to produce acetylcholine. Most obvious and easy to get at, however, is the enzyme **cholinesterase**, the essential function of which is to break down acetylcholine.

As noted above, in a crude interference with brain function, usual medical treatment of Alzheimer's focuses on inhibiting this enzyme. All three of the main drugs currently approved to treat Alzheimer's in America are aimed at maintaining acetylcholine levels. Tacrine, donepezil, and rivastigmine all act by inhibiting cholinesterase.[19] These drugs, however, do nothing to attack the root causes of acetylcholine decline, or slow the loss of hippocampal cells, or prevent the build-up of abnormal proteins. So it is not surprising they provide only temporary relief of symptoms and do not stop or reverse even the mildest of Alzheimer's.

The drugs miss the boat because they do not tackle the most basic

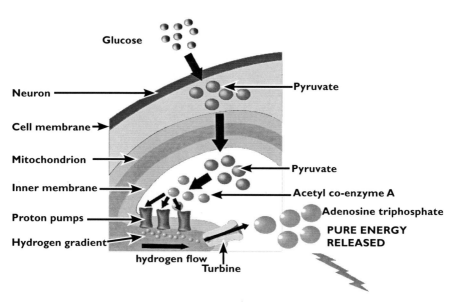

Figure 9.9. Glycolytic pathway.

mechanism of acetylcholine decline. To understand it, we have to go back to Chapter 4 and the decline of glucose metabolism. The biochemistry is a bit of a brain strain, so it bears repeating here. Glucose metabolism, or the **glycolytic pathway** as it is called (Figure 9.9), produces about two molecules of acetyl-coenzyme A for every 38 molecules of glucose. If glucose metabolism declines by half, as it does between ages 25 and 75, then acetyl-coenzyme A drops by half.

Acetyl-coenzyme A is also a key precursor of acetylcholine in the brain.[18] So, if it declines, then acetylcholine declines also. Our primary task in preventing acetylcholine decline is to maintain normal production of acetyl-coenzyme A lifelong. We covered the program we use to do this in chapter 5 - 7.

Multiple Nutrients Required

In order to protect the brain from the six causes of damage that develop into Alzheimer's, we have to use every one of the nutrients examined throughout this book. In short, the prevention of Alzheimer's requires a full brain program, such as I have explained in all the previous chapters put together. It may seem a lot, but is really a small price to pay to keep your cognition intact lifelong. It is summarized in Chapter 10.

Should you be wavering at all the trouble and expense, it bears repeating that current health policies cannot protect you. The massive health benefits and astronomical savings in medical and business costs that would result from instituting brain protective programs to protect the population from Alzheimer's, are beyond the intellectual grasp of current policy makers.

Don't be too hard on them. Because of political pressures, many of these folk are concerned only with actions that will benefit their positions while they are in office. National vaccination cost untold billions, but it worked fast. The political benefits were obvious. Unlike national vaccination, saving brains is a 40–50 year process. Politicians do not yet remain in authority that long.

Protecting the human brain will get the recognition it deserves. We lost one president because Alzheimer's was not detected early enough because the science was not there. Now, with the combination of new brain science and the increasing age levels of our politicians at all levels of government, there is a growing sense of self-preservation regarding cognition. I venture to predict that, within 20 years, strategies similar to those outlined here will be considered as important in health policy as vaccination or antibiotics. As study piles upon study, it is becoming clear beyond ignoring that, if we lose our brains at the present rate, the aging populations of America and Canada simply cannot stand. Until this disastrous trend is fully accepted and acted upon by government, you have to protect yourself.

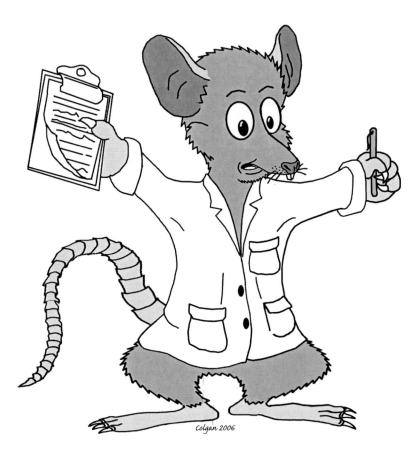

"Who could care less about the War on Terror. I'm
voting for the candidate who will save my brain."

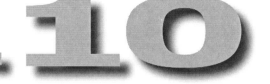

The Brain Program

We have examined a small, but I hope representative, sample of the evidence that the mitochondria, energy-producing structures in our neurons, are subjected to free radical damage from about 5% of the oxygen they use to perform their function, which escapes control. As a result of this damage, from about age 20 to 60 (70 if you are lucky in choosing your parents or smart in choosing your lifestyle), our production of adenosine triphosphate (ATP) declines by about half. Not only do we lose half our physical and mental energy, but the protective "electric fences," that is the trans-membrane potentials that keep harmful chemicals out of our neurons, lose half their power. By about age 35-45, they no longer work as well as they should. By age 60-70, they no longer work properly at all, causing detrimental effects on brain function, memory, and new learning, and affecting every other system and organ in your body.

When the trans-membrane potentials decline, chemicals such as glutamate then punch "holes" through receptors, allowing substances such as calcium to enter the cell and produce deadly free radicals, such as **peroxynitrite**, which progressively add to the brain damage.

As we examined in Chapters 1-4, the oxidation damage to mitochondria also causes rancidity of lipids and chronic inflammation in the brain as we age. Additionally, it disrupts portions of our DNA code, so that key essential proteins in the body accumulate errors.

We have also looked briefly at recent research showing that most degenerative disease of the human brain, including Alzheimer's, Parkinson's, and other subdivisions of the brain damage of usual aging, involve certain structures in our ancient midbrain. Research suggests that these structures evolved first as the brain of early reptiles, probably more than 300 million years ago. Today that brain, or something very like it, still exists in modern crocodiles. In us, as in them, the R-complex of brain structures mediates powerful emotions of fear, anger, and territoriality, which still, far too often control human behavior.

The research herein indicates that these structures are less robust than the largest part of our brain, the most recently evolved majority of our cerebral cortex, and are more subject to the ravages of our culturally mandated elected, long-as-possible lifetime.

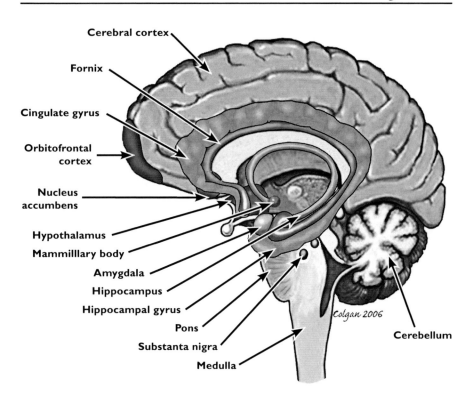

Figure 10.1. A review of the main structures involved in brain degeneration. They are:
Hippocampus and its surrounding essential structures for formation of memories.
Substantia nigra, essential for precise movements, coordination, and balance.
Amygdala, a mediating structure for anger, fear, and anxiety.
Above these we have noted the more recently evolved:
Cingulate gyrus, an essential structure for attention and cognitive processing.
Orbitofrontal cortex, an essential structure for decision making.

From Chapters 2-4, we know that the most affected brain structures, especially the hippocampus and the substantia nigra, degenerate in almost all of us at a rate of 4-8% per decade from about age 25. For many people, the disastrous effects on cognition and memory, emotions, and physical capacity begin to show in four to five decades, that is by the time they are 65-75. In the interim, the brain damage also promotes many other bodily diseases, diseases that often claim the host before the mind clouds.

As life expectancy continues to extend, an ever growing proportion of our population will be victims of mental degeneration to the point of incapacity to care for themselves. By 2030, the burden of care will be such that no business expansions or industrial growth, even at triple the current rates in America, can possibly support it.

The current official approach to degenerative brain disease is to pretend it doesn't exist, until the individual presents with undeniable symptoms. It's not so long ago that medicine used to pretend that infection, which killed up to 50% of hospital patients, did not exist because you cannot see the living organisms, germs, floating in the air. Louis Pasteur first suggested it in 1865, and Joseph Lister proved it when he completely prevented sepsis with a carbolic spray at the Glasgow Royal Infirmary in Scotland in 1869.[1]

We are at the same bulwark today with degenerative brain disease. Medical authorities ignore the invisible disease, quietly destroying our brains. By the time of diagnosis, when symptoms are obvious, all that is left to do is palliative symptomatic care until death.

Consider teeth. We spend billions on check-ups and repair. We have been taught very well to do so. Yet you can live comfortably with numerous lost teeth or even none at all. You can put off going to the dentist for years, and still have your teeth repaired. You cannot live comfortably with even 25% of lost cells in the hippocampus and substantia nigra of your brain. You cannot put off brain degeneration. It waits for no one. It damages every organ and system in your body and it is irreparable.

It is my contention herein, that we should focus our medical efforts on prevention of damage to the hippocampus, the substantia nigra, and associated structures, at least to the same degree that we currently focus on the prevention of damage to our teeth.

The Current Brain Program

Our current Brain Program at the Colgan Institute is briefly reviewed in Chapters 5-9. It is an audacious effort to use the huge advances in brain research to maintain human brain function lifelong. This book is my effort to present a brief summary of the information publicly, in an easily understood format, so that you, the reader, may seek the scientific references for yourself and decide whether our thesis is sound.

Because of the huge individual differences in brain function, and because I have not been able to meet you personally and review your history and lifestyle, whatever use you may make of the information herein is, as always, at your own choice and sole risk. Nevertheless, I feel confident in the science, and optimistic that it will be implemented in public health policy within my lifetime by sound and far-sighted leadership. This book is only a tiny bugle call. When the charge of the new brain science occurs, medicine will change utterly.

The following tables are self-explanatory and summarize tables given in Chapters 5-7.

Table 10.1. Prevention of Chronic Inflammation of the Brain

Substance	Range of Daily intake
Aspirin	325 – 650 mg
Turmeric	
Curcumin	150 – 300 mg
Xanthorrizol 8% extract	150 – 300 mg
Beta-tumerone 8% extract	150 – 300 mg
Piperine	250 – 50 mg
Cinnamon (powdered bark)	1.0 – 3.0 grams
Ginger (5% gingerol extract)	400 – 800 mg
Cloves (powdered)	1.0 – 2.0 grams
Cayenne (dilute capsaicin)	250 – 500 mg
Docosahexaenoic acid	500 – 1000 mg

Table 10.2. Mitochondrial Protection

Substance	Range of Daily Intake
R+ lipoic acid	200 – 800 mg
Acetyl-l-carnitine[*†]	500 – 2500 mg
N-acetyl-cysteine	200 – 400 mg
Idebenone	200 – 400 mg
Selegiline[*†*]	1.0 – 6.0 mg
CDP-choline	500 – 1000 mg

Taken in divided doses, half in a.m., half at noon, with food.
*† We do not take acetyl-L-carnitine or selegiline after 3 pm, because they stimulate the function of "get-up-and-go" neurotransmitters, dopamine and acetylcholine.
* Selegiline Use: We individualize selegiline by numerous criteria, but the most important are Biological Age and sex. See table in Chapter 5.

Table 10.3. Prevention of Excess Nitric Oxide Production

Substance	Range of Daily Intake
Genestein[*]	10 – 50 mg
Allicin[*]	50 – 150 mg
Gingko[*]	200 – 500 mg
Silymarin[*]	150 – 450 mg
Aminoguanidine	150 – 300 mg
Aspirin	150 – 650 mg
Docosohexaenoic acid [†]	500 – 1000 mg
Phenyl-butyl nitrone (PBN)	Not yet commercially available in an effective supplement form

* Extractions are not given for some herbals because of wide variations in chemistry of commercial products.
† This amount is in addition to the DHA in Table 10.1.

Coffee Break

In addition to the tables alone, to help prevent the Parkinson's complex of diseases, we use coffee. The name comes from the ancient Arabic *gahweh* meaning "gives strength." The stimulant effects of coffee and its effects on clarity of thought, have been known for thousands of years. As always, it is the dose which makes the poison or the medicine. We examined the research in Chapter 8 that more than three cups per day have a less and less beneficial effect in preventing Parkinson's. And excess coffee is known to cause delirium and hallucinations, and withdrawal from habitual excess coffee is known to cause severe depression.[2]

You have to have the right coffee. The berries (usually called "beans") of *Coffea robusta*, which is used to make most instant coffees and diner coffee, have a much different chemical structure than "real" coffee. Real coffee is made solely of *Coffea arabica* berries. Grind organic fair-trade beans (berries) yourself, for each pot, and brew a daily cupful of delight. Your brain will repay the kindness lifelong.

Tea Time

Then there's tea. Both black (roasted) and green teas contain polyphenols, the latter with at least twice the quantity. One big surprise of the recent research we examined in Chapter 9, is confirmation of the potency of polyphenols in preventing damage to neurons by beta-amyloid, one of the major gremlins in Alzheimer's.

Even better, and much higher in polyphenols, is real dark chocolate (organic, of course), that is chocolate made from the dried seeds of the cocoa tree, *Theobroma cacao*. Named by the great botanist Carolus Linnaeus, who gave us our current classification of plants way back in the 18th century, it means "food of the gods." It certainly is. Nice to know it helps to protect us from Alzheimer's.

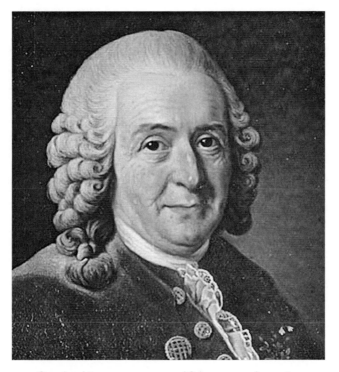

Carolus Linnaeus, greatest 18th-century botanist, who gave us our modern taxonomy of plants.

Flee the City

There is so much. We have not covered the beneficial effect of physical exercise. We have not even touched on the beneficial effects of deliberate, study and new learning lifelong. We have not discussed the large detrimental effects on the brain, of loss of estrogen in women at menopause and loss of testosterone in men at viripause. All are covered in part in previous books from the Colgan Institute.[3-5]

But there is one more topic I must cover herein - city life. Cities are now far too polluted for long-term health of the human brain. No matter what supplements you take, you cannot overcome the thousands of man-made chemicals in the air, against which your genome has evolved negligible defenses because it never encountered them in its evolution.

With high-tech communications and business systems today, it is feasible to leave cities and live in clean air and drink clean water far from the *madding crowd*. Better than going through the vast research on city pollution, I would like to present just one potent example, the very best sort of scientific example because it involves real people living in a part of a city with a hugely accelerated concentration of air pollution. That place is Ground Zero.

On 11 September 2001, the destruction of the World Trade Center in New York created urban environmental pollution of previously unknown magnitude in the United States. Asbestos (from the asbestos/concrete mix cladding the walls) lead, mercury, benzene, polychlorinated biphenyls, dioxins, and vast concentrations of multiple volatile solvents made the air unfit to breathe for many months afterwards.[6] Yet, on instructions from the White House to downplay the environmental danger, on September 16, 2001, the head of the Environmental Protection Agency, Christie Todd Whitman, released a public statement:

> *I am glad to reassure the people of New York… that their air is safe to breathe, their water is safe to drink.*[7]

By 2002 more than 10,000 people who worked at or near Ground Zero, or lived within a mile of it, became ill. Today Mount Sinai Medical Center is monitoring the health of more than 71,000 people thought to have become ill from Ground Zero exposure. The rates of Alzheimer's and Parkinson's in these people are expected to be gigantic. There are two class-action lawsuits brought against the EPA and the American government, representing more than 12,000 people who have become ill or died from the Ground Zero pollution.

Nine police officers who worked at Ground Zero have brain cancer or have died of brain cancer.[8] Thirty-four-year-old New York detective James Zadroga, who toiled daily at the site, died with high levels of mercury in his brain.

As I write, news media are reporting that the immunity against prosecution afforded public officials has been withdrawn from former EPA head Christie Todd Whitman. It will still be a long road to justice, however, too late for the thousands of people who cannot work, or even think clearly enough any more to defend themselves against bureaucracy.

You may remember, I hope you remember, *Minamata disease*, a brain-destroying condition caused by methylmercury, first discovered in 1956 in Minamata Bay in Japan. Autopsies showed huge destruction of the brain, including the cerebral cortex itself. That particular pattern of brain degeneration is now recognized (after death) in numerous cases world-wide.[9,10] People who lived or worked at or near the World Trade Center will probably also show a particular pattern of brain destruction, that may well warrant the name Ground Zero disease.

So, you don't live near Ground Zero, so what's it to do with your brain? The Ground Zero example is simply an accelerated form of the brain pollution that is happening to all big city dwellers. The exact same toxins are in the air of every city in America, though in much smaller concentrations. Too small to damage you? There are no safe levels for lead, mercury, benzene, or many other brain poisons. Do not expect the health authorities to protect your brain from pollution. You have to learn to protect yourself.

A Personal Note

When we worked with Hollywood celebrities in the 1980s, we had a Colgan Institute clinic on Sunset Boulevard in Los Angeles and lived nearby, a stone's throw from the major film studios. Yet we were always advising the stars to leave the city, and several did, much to the chagrin of studio bosses because of the increased problems of travel and communication. One day, studio head Bob Shapiro confronted me with, "Well why are you living here?" I thought about it seriously for two weeks while I dealt with necessary notice to staff and wind-down, locked my office on the Friday night – and left permanently for Encinitas, near San Diego, which had pretty clean air at that time. My attorney, Roy Bell, rang me hot and bothered on Monday, telling me that I had ruined his Saturday golf game. He had received a call on the course from a celebrity client demanding to know where I was. "I quit," I told him. I still remember his exact admonition. "Are you crazy? You just ruined a multi-million dollar business!"

He was probably right. Hollywood rarely gives the "trades" second chances. But, after half a century of adulthood, my brain still works fine and dandy.

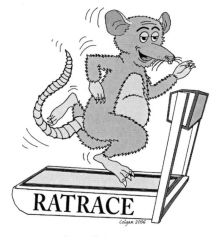

Get off the rat race.

Study the references well and decide for yourself whether or not to protect your brain. And if you do, find a good physician to assist you and monitor whatever you decide to do. There is a list of anti-aging physicians, some of whom specialize in protecting the human brain. You can access it at www.worldhealth.net I wish you luck in finding a wise one. I also wish you 100 years of a clear mind and a happy heart.

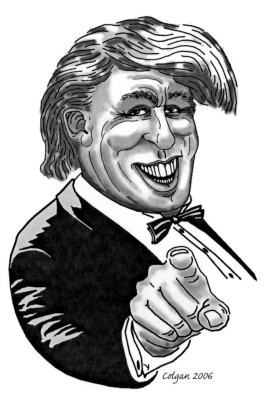

"I took the Brain Program. Look what it did for me!!"

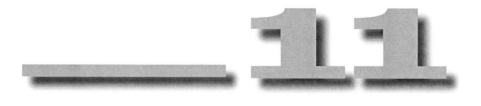

A Quiet Mind

We have examined some of the recent science indicating that specific chemicals and lifestyle practices can protect the **structure** of your brain against the ravages of time. But the chemistry does not address one of the largest large causes of brain degeneration, in fact the biggest single cause of illness throughout the Westernized world - **emotional disorder**. Unlike the physical structure of the brain, there is no chemical protection for damaging emotion.

As we saw in Chapter 6, needless fear, anxiety, and anger generate excess nitric oxide in the brain, with consequent damage to cells in the hippocampus, our essential mediating structure for memory. In Chapter 3, we examined research showing that fear and anger also damage the mitochondria, and reduce the supply of ATP. Worse, these emotions, which stem from our reptilian mid-brain, cause our fast, excitatory neurotransmitter glutamate to run wild, punching "holes" in cell membranes which cause chemical leaks, and consequent formation of the deadly free radical peroxynitrite. These events occur on a daily basis in the average person who chooses to live in our tightly packed urban communities, where personal space is measured in inches, yet our brains remain those of a hunter, who evolved in sparsely populated countryside. [1,2]

More than 30 million Americans and 3 million Canadians currently gobble gazillions of antidepressant, antipsychotic, and anti-anxiety prescription medications in vain efforts to keep negative emotions under control. In the US, use of anti-depressants more than tripled between 1990 and 2005.   One in every ten people you see walking down the mall   now takes medication to relieve the symptoms of emotional distress. Mostly these are selective-serotonin-reuptake inhibitors (SSRI), which keep the brain high in serotonin, the neurotransmitter of sleep.[3,4]   Short-term, these chemical straightjackets relieve emotional distress by numbing the mind, just as novocaine numbs the pain of an abscessed tooth. But, like novocaine, these pills and potions do nothing to cure the condition.

As we saw in Chapter 2, emotional distress arises because each of us owns a mid-brain that evolved under a completely different environment, an environment in which if you did not fight or flee immediately, you were killed and eaten. And, of course, there are still real threats to our physical well-being.   Fire burns flesh regardless of thought. Unlike fire, however, most life events today are not inherently damaging. They become so only when we attach negative emotions to them.   Cool water can raise real burns, if the victim is led to fear it is boiling.   Such is the power of negative emotions to damage your physical structure.

Fear is a major culprit. Yet fear does not exist in any object or situation. It has no physical existence at all. Fear is purely an emotional construction you build in your mind. Whenever you become afraid, you have frightened yourself. Consequently, emotional disorder can never be cured by drugs, nutrients, surgery, or any medical intervention, because it is rooted in your memory and triggered by your environment. It can be cured only by making changes to your mind.

To make these changes by yourself is difficult. To indicate one way, I want to share with you a brief look at the method we use, which has enabled many folk to remove emotional distress from their lives. To do so is far more valuable to your health, your well-being, and your brain than any nutritional regime, any medical treatment, any doctor, any other approach to life. We call it - **growing the quiet mind.**

How Emotional Disorder Occurs

Many of the emotional constructions we attach to life events, occur beneath the surface of consciousness. Thoughts invade the mind at such a rapid rate, that we can give to each barely time to recognize its passing. Yet each thought excites emotional circuits in the brain that reverberate long after it is gone. These emotional residues often become permanent memories.

A lifelong irrational fear of spiders for example, can follow a single unpleasant experience of one crawling innocently into your ear. The neural stimulation from such negative emotional memories, affects hypothalamic-limbic-pituitary circuits in the mid-brain, and disturbs the autonomic nervous system that controls all your housekeeping functions, from heartbeat, to gut reactions, to elimination. It also damages your immune system, your hormones, and your brain.[5]

If your past life is predominantly happy, the emotional residues of positive thoughts accumulate in your memory to form an underlying current of **eu-stress** so named by the great Canadian physician Hans Selye. While working with Dr. Selye in the 1970's, I learned how eu-stress shapes the mind to cultivate a confident and resilient personality, resistant to negative emotions. In concert, eu-stress promotes physical and mental health, strength and growth. I also learned how the emotional residues of predominantly negative thoughts, accumulate to form an underlying current of **dis-stress**. Distress cultivates an anxious and fearful personality, which promotes physical and mental illness, weakness and premature aging. We all live at habitual points on the continuum of eu-stress and distress.

Those of us who live towards the pole of emotional distress, tend to be chronically physically sickly, and find it difficult to pursue our goals in life. Distressed folk find it almost impossible to progress towards the four universal life goals of: excellence in work, closeness

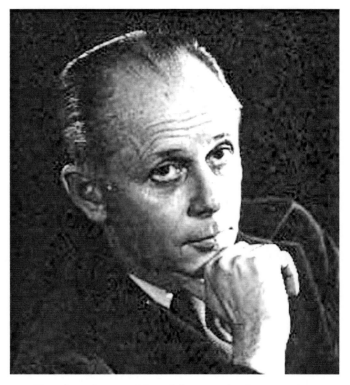

Canadian physician Hans Selye was the first to relate emotional stress to particular circuits in the brain.

in personal relationships, compassion for those around you, and nobility in everything you do. Habitual emotional distress also makes difficult any enduring steps to change it. Each step outside the comfort zone of "woe is me," is akin to giving up a teddy bear, and requires the outside support of a wise person who is high on the eu-stress pole of life. These folk are hard to find.

The Way of the Quiet Mind

To ease the path we have developed the **Quiet Mind Program**. Quiet mind is a state in which the negative emotional baggage of your past can be viewed dispassionately for what it is — destructive emotional memories constructed by your past reactions to unpleasant situations. Just as you have placed each one of these memories, so the quiet mind can show you how to remove it.

The source of our method is Zen Buddhism. This ideology has been developed continuously for the last 2,500 years. It is useful to know how it began. Contrary to popular belief, Zen is not Japanese in origin. It is derived from the Sanskrit "Dyana" which began in India with the birth of Siddhartha Gautama in 563 BC. He founded Buddhism.

Over the next 10 centuries, this obscure Hindu sect grew rapidly and spread to Tibet and China, where Dyana was translated into Chinese as "Ch'an". Under the T'ang dynasty (618-906 AD), Ch'an Buddhism flourished among artists and intellectuals. During the Sung dynasty (960-1276 AD), it spread to all classes, and became the dominant influence on Chinese culture and education.

By the 11th century, Chinese monks visiting Japan, and Japanese monks studying in China, had exported Ch'an Buddhism to Japan. "Ch'an" became "Zen" in English because that is how it is pronounced in Japanese. The nearest English word is "contemplation".[6,7]

From what is now called "1st century AD", another obscure sect grew from the teachings of Jesus of Nazareth to become "Christianity." Widely adopted by the Romans who ruled most of the Western world at that time, it became based in Rome as "Roman Catholicism." Recognizing the power of its ideology, Rome replaced the failing power of its armies with Catholicism, as a better way to control its Empire.

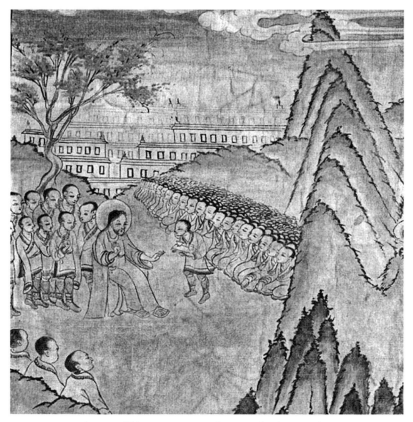

Ancient Tibetan painting frequently depicted in historical texts as Jesus teaching in Tibet.

To achieve acceptance of Catholicism, Rome had to rewrite history so as to integrate its ideology with the diverse "pagan" religions and their deities of the countries they ruled. They had to raise Jesus from the status of a mortal prophet to that of a deity. Consequently, they had to eliminate the Gospels that spoke of the 17 years of travels of Jesus to India and Tibet, from age 13 to 30 to study and preach Buddhism,[8-11] which was then considered in Europe an ideology of barbarians.

Given the power that Rome achieved by deification of Jesus – to "the Christ," "the Son of God", it is understandable that Christian ideologies continue to do everything possible to dispute the history that Jesus studied Buddhism for most of his life, and based his ministry in Israel upon it. And indeed, most of the real history is lost in time, with much speculation and little evidence, as is the real history of the New Testament, which, nevertheless, is currently accepted without question by many people

The recent re-discovery of the Judas Gospel, has caused many people to reconsider the Bible as a man-made and many times altered document, and more subject to human frailties than we would like to believe. I include a mention of the history here, only to indicate that our method of achieving a quiet mind is not based on some esoteric oriental ideology because of its current popularity in the West, but on the dominant ideology on Earth, an ideology which is probably the basis of both Buddhism and Christianity.

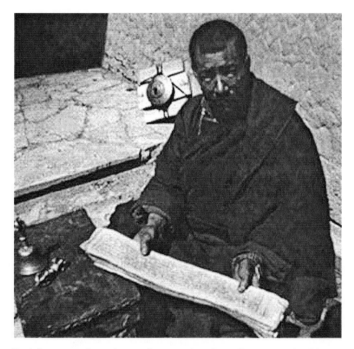

Buddhist monk with scroll recording Jesus's stay at the Hemis
monastery at Ladakh on the border between India and Tibet.

The reason we focus on the Zen sect and its practices, is that its
isolation in Japan protected it to some extent from the corruption
of competing ideologies, corruption that has been rife throughout
the Christian world from the Dark Ages of the Inquisition until
the present. Should you feel uneasy at my criticism of Christianity,
remember it has not changed since the unfortunate women of
Salem were put to death as witches in "enlightened" America, all in
the name of a Christian God. Fortunately the Buddhist/Christian
ideology has survived these corruptions, so that we can live together
in a civilized manner, hopefully in joy, love and compassion.

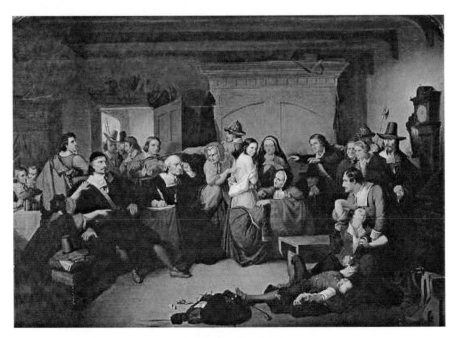

Salem witch trials

Since 1200 AD, Zen has been continuously refined in Japan, and has exerted profound influence on the development of Japanese culture. Practitioners offer two main methods of advancement. The Soto sect (Farmer zen) favors regular meditation to promote a gradual dawning of insight. The Rinzai sect (Warrior zen) favors flashes of insight that occur by regular contemplation of koans (apparently illogical statements). Both sects agree on the necessity to achieve a quiet mind, which they call **mushin**. The best I can do to explain mushin in English, is a mind free from artifice, distraction, obstruction and inhibition.

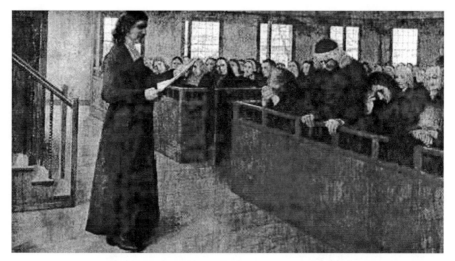

Recantation of his judgements of witchcraft
by judge Samuel Sewell after the Salem trials.

The central practice of Zen, called **zazen**, involves sitting for a period each day in meditation. From our experience with thousands of athletes, and folk seeking answers to aging and illness, who come unbidden to the Colgan Institute, we have found zazen difficult for Westerners. Most of us are brought up to crave external stimulation. We are taught to revere busy-ness (business), and live under the illusion that solutions to many problems can be acquired immediately, like instant mashed potato. To sit for a period each day, apparently doing nothing, for years, seems appropriate only for the old and feeble. In 1996, we resolved to find an easier way.

Steps to A Quiet Mind

Over the last ten years, we have developed a method of contemplation more appropriate to Western culture. We teach people to meditate while busily in action, doing repetitive daily tasks, tasks that require little thought, such as tending a garden, jogging, and especially, exercising in the Colgan Power Program.

In initial stages, with each repetition of the task, you are taught to focus on your center and what we call Three-Part Breathing. Then, after some weeks of practice, you are taught to focus on greater and greater refinement of form and movement. Then, after some months of practice, you focus on performing the same motions with less and less effort.

We use this method for every set of every exercise at advanced levels of the Power Program. We teach athletes, and folk seeking extended healthy lives, to incorporate greater and greater **relaxation, coordination, rhythm** and **fluidity** into all their movements. Gradually, they become able to exert maximum force with very little effort or movement at all. Consciously doing the movement eventually becomes the movement doing itself.

Once you have reached this level of **quiet mind**, you can step back from your body and observe yourself. The unique causes of your emotional stress, the blocks to achieving what you desire in life, become more and more obvious, and easier and easier to confront and form a plan to eliminate.

From this position, you can learn to do many life activities in **quiet mind**, which prevents new negative emotional memories, and new blocks to progress from forming. The ultimate goal is to live every moment of life in this state, free from the damage of fear, anxiety, anger, hatred, and depression. Gradually, your mind becomes emptied of emotional clutter, allowing clearer and clearer thought.

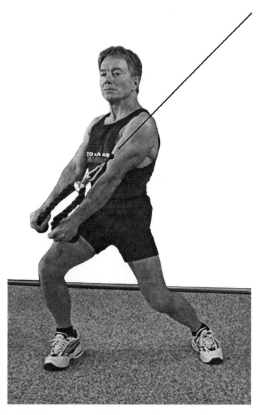

Michael Colgan at age 67 in meditation while exercising.

Clear human thought has no bounds. That which you can imagine strongly enough you can achieve. But you need a mind free from negative emotions in order to focus sharply on the path. Adopt the **Quiet Mind Program**, and join me in the journey to perfect your capacity for the joyous emotions of love and compassion. Achieve your unique and bountiful place on this Earth, midst the beauty and growth and rhythms of Nature, in trees and mountains and oceans, and the perpetual rising of the sun.

References

Chapter 1: Brain Strain

1. Calabrese V, et al. NO synthase and NO-dependent signal pathways in brain aging and neurodegenerative disorders, the role of oxidant/antioxidant balance. *Neurochem Res*, 2000; 25:1315-1341.

2. National Institute of Mental Health. Prevalence of dementia and other neurodegenerative diseases. 2002. www.nimh.nih.gov. Accessed, 20 August 2006.

3. US Dept. of Health & Human Services. Progress Report on Alzheimer's Disease; 2000. www.alzheimers.org/pubs *NIH Publication* No. 00-4859.

4. National Parkinson's Foundation. *Parkinson's Disease.* 1999 .www.parkinson.org/ encarta. Accessed 21, August 2006.

5. Perlmutter D. Functional therapies in neurodegenerative disease. *J Appl Nutr,* 1999; 51:3-13.

6. Grossman LI. Mitochondrial mutations and human disease. *Environ Mol Mutagen*, 1995; 25:(Suppl 26):30-37.

7. Shigenaga MK, et al. Oxidative damage and mitochondrial decay in aging. *Proc Natl Acad Sci USA.* 1994; 91:10771-10778.

8. Bittles AH. Evidence for and against the causal involvement of mitochondrial DNA mutation in mammalian aging. *Mutat Res*, 1992; 275:217-225.

9. Meier-Ruge W, et al. What is primary and what secondary for amyloid deposition in Alzheimer's. *Ann NY Acad Sci*, 1994; 719:230-237.

10. Finnegan MJ, et al. The sick building syndrome: prevalence studies. *Brit Med J,* 1984; 289: 1573-1575.

11. Semchuk KM, et al. Parkinson's disease and exposure to agricultural work and pesticide chemicals. *Neurology,* 1992; 42: 1328-1335.

12. Baldi A, et al. Association between Parkinson's disease and exposure to pesticides in south-western France. *Neuroepidemiology,* 2003: 305-310.

13. Harman D. Alzheimer's disease: role of aging in pathogenesis. *Ann NY Acad Sci,* 2002; 959:384-395.

14. Beckman JS. Peroxynitrite versus hydroxyl radical: The role of nitric oxide in superoxide dependent cerebral injury. *Ann NY Acad Sci,* 1994; 738:69-75.

15. Barbu A, et al. Cytokine-induced apoptosis and necrosis are preceded by disruption of the mitochondrial membrane potential. *Mol Cell Endocrinol,* 2002; 190:75-82.

16. Colgan M. *Hormonal Health.* Vancouver: Apple Publishing, 1996.

17. Shaw CE, et al. Progress in the pathogenesis of amyotrophic lateral sclerosis. *Curr Neurol Neurosci,* 2001; 1:69-76.

18. Zenon MM, et al. Mutant Huntington enhances excitotoxic cell death. *Moll Cell Neurosci,* 2001; 17:41-53.

19. Paty DW, Ebars GC (Eds). *Multiple Sclerosis,* Philadelphia:FA Davis, 1998.

Chapter 2: In the Beginning

1. Ferrier D, et al. The amphioxus Hox cluster. *Evolution and Development,* 2000: 2:284-293.

2. Fastovsky DE, Weishampel, F. *The Evolution and Extinction of the Dinosaurs.* New York: Cambridge University Press, 1996.

3. Milne-Edwards A, Grandidier A. *Histoire Physique, Naturelle et Politique de Madagasar,* Vol. 9, Paris 1875.

4. Johanson D, Edgar B. *From Lucy to Language.* New York: Simon and Shuster, 1996.

5. Hurford JF, et al (Eds). *Approaches to the Evolution of Language.* Cambridge: Cambridge University Press, 1998.

6. Dunbar RIM. Coevolution of neocortical size, group size, and language in humans. *Behavioral and Brain Sci,* 1993; 16:681-735.

Chapter 3: Brains at Risk

1. MacLean P. *The Triune Brain in Evolution.* New York: Plenum, 1990.

2. Gall FJ, Spurzheim JG. *Anatomie et Physionomie du Systeme Nerveux en General et du Cerveau en Particulier.* Vols. 1-4. Paris: F Schoell, 1810-1818.

3. Skabaneck P, McCormick J. *Follies and Fallacies in Medicine.* New York: Prometheus, 1990.

4. Sabbatini RM. The history of brain localization. *Brain and Mind,* March, 1997.

5. Le Master JR, Kummings DD. *Walt Whitman: An Encyclopedia.* New York: Garland,1998.

6. Nolte J. *The Human Brain: An Introduction to its Functional Anatomy.* London: Mosby, 2001.

7. US National Institute on Drug Abuse, National Institute of Health. *Mind Over Matter.* www.nida.gov/MOM. June 2002.

8. Kandel E, Schwatz J. *Principles of Neural Science.* New York: Appleton and Lange, 2000.

9. Pepe C, Hammond L. *Reversing Multiple Sclerosis.* London: Hampton Roads, 2001.

10. Colgan M. *Hormonal Health.* Vancouver: Apple Publishing, 1996.

Chapter 4: Mitochondrial Decay

1. de Grey AD. *The Mitochondrial Free Radical Theory of Aging.* Georgetown TX: Landes Bioscience, 1999.

2. Hagen TM. *Mitochondrial decay in aging.* Paper presented at the 29th Annual ISOM Conference. April 6-9 2000, Vancouver, B.C.

3. Hagen TM, et al. (R+) alpha lipoic acid – supplemented old rats have improved mitochondrial function, decreased oxidative damage and increased metabolic rate. *FASEB*, 1999; 13:411-418.

4. Lee HA, Hughes DA. Alpha-lipoic acid modulates NF-kappa-B activity in human monocytic cells by direct interaction with DNA. *Exp Gerontol,* 2002; 37:401-410.

5. Hawking S. *The Universe in a Nutshell.* New York, NY:Bantam Books, 2001.

6. Gribbin J, Gribbin M. *Stardust.Supernovae and Life – the Cosmic Connection.* Massachusetts, Yale University Press, 2000.

7. Mattson MP, et al. Modification of brain aging and neurodegenerative disorders by genes, diet, and behavior. *Physiol Rev,* 2002; 82:637-672.

8. Liu J, et al. Delaying brain mitochondrial decay and aging with mitochondrial antioxidants and metabolites. *Ann N Y Acad Sci,* 2002; 959:133-166.

9. Bittles AH. Evidence for and against the causal involvement of mitochondria DNA mutation in mammalian aging. *Mutat Res,* 1992; 275:217-225.

Chapter 5: Saving Your Mitochondria

1. Liu J, et al. Memory loss in old rats is associated with brain mitochondrial decay and RNA/DNA oxidation: partial reversal by feeding acetyl-l-carnitine and/or R-alpha-lipoic acid. *Proc Natl Acad Sci USA,* 2002; 99:2356-2361.

2. Knight JA. Reactive oxygen species and the neurodegenerative disorders. *Ann Clin Lab Sci,* 1997; 27:11-25.

3. Calabrese V, et al. Mitochondrial Involvement in brain function and dysfunction: relevance to aging, neurodegenerative disorders and longevity. *Neurochem Res,* 2001; 26:739-764.

4. Grossman LI. Mitochondrial mutations and human disease. *Environ Mol Mutagen,* 1995; 26:30-37.

5. Schapira AH, et al. Mitochondrial function in neurodegeneration and aging. *Mutat Res,* 1992; 275:133-143.

6. Harman D. Aging: a theory based on free radical and radiation chemistry. *J Gerontol,* 1956; 11:298-300.

7. Lee HA, et al. Alpha-lipoic acid modulates NF-kappa-B activity in human monocytic cells by direct interaction with DNA. *Exp Gerontol,* 2002; 37:401-410.

8. Harman D. The biologic clock: the mitochondria? *J Am Geriatr Soc,* 1972; 20:145-147.

9. Colgan M. *Sports Nutrition Guide.* Vancouver,: Apple Publishing, 2002.

10. Colgan M. *Nutrition for Champions.* Vancouver: Science Books, 2007.

11. Packer L, et al. *Handbook of Antioxidants.* New York: Marcel Dekker, 1996.

12. Lockhart B, et al. Inhibition of L-homocysteic acid and buthionine sulphoximine-mediated neurotoxicity in rat embryonic neuronal cultures with alpha-lipoic acid enantiomers. *Brain Res,* 2000; 855(2):292-297.

13. Suh JH, et al. Dietary supplementation with (R)-alpha-lipoic acid reverses the age-related accumulation of iron and depletion of antioxidants in the rat cerebral cortex. *Redox Rep,* 2005; 10(1):52-60

14. Hagen T, et al. R-alpha lipoic acid-supplemented old rats have improved mitochondrial function, decreased oxidative damage, and increased metabolic rate. *FASEB J,* 1999; 13:411-418.

15. Frolich L, et al. (r)-, but not (s)-alpha lipoic acid stimulates deficient brain pyruvate dehydrogenase complex in vascular dementia, but not in Alzheimer dementia. *J Neural Transm,* 2004; 111(3):295-310.

16. Schulz JB, et al. Glutathione, oxidative stress and neurodegeneration. *Eur J*

Biochem, 2000; 267(16):4904-4911.

17. Sian J, et al. Alterations in glutathione levels in Parkinson's disease and other neurodegenerative disorders affecting basal ganglia. *Ann Neurol,* 1994; 36(3):348-355.

18. Singh I, et al. Cytokine-mediated induction of ceramide is redox-sensitive. Implications to proinflammatory cytokine-mediated apoptosis in demyelinating diseases. *J Biol Chem,* 1998; 273(32):20354-20362.

19. Lin J, et al. Effect of R-(+)-alpha-lipoic acid on experimental diabetic retinopathy. *Diabetologia,* 2006; 49(5):1089-1096.

20. 20.Voloboueva LA, et al. (R)-alpha-lipoic acid protects retinal pigment epithelial cells from oxidative damage. *Invest Ophthalmol Vis Sci,* 2005; 46(11):4301-4310.

21. Henriksen EJ, et al. Exercise training and antioxidants: relief from oxidative stress and insulin resistance. *Exerc Sport Sci Rev,* 2003; 31(2): 79-84.

22. Colgan M. *You Can Prevent Cancer.* Vancouver: Apple Publishing, 2007.

23. Hang YS, et al. *Free Rad Biol Med,* 1999; 26:685-694.

24. Ames BN, Lin J. Delaying the mitochondrial decay of aging with acetylcarnitine. *Ann N Y Acad Sci,* 2004; 1033:108-116.

25. Suh JH, et al. (R)-alpha-lipoic acid reverses the age-related loss in GSH redox status in post-mitotic tissues: evidence for increased cysteine requirement for GSH synthesis. *Arch Biochem Biophys,* 2004; 423(1):126-135.

26. Miquel J. Can antioxidant diet supplementation protect against age-related mitochondrial damage? *Ann N Y Acad Sci,* 2002; 959:508-516.

27. Colgan M. *Hormonal Health.* Vancouver, Apple Publishing, 1996.

28. Liu J, et al. Delaying brain mitochondrial decay and aging with mitochondrial antioxidants and metabolites. *Ann N Y Acad Sci,* 2002; 959:133-166.

29. Hagen TM, et al. Feeding acetyl-L-carnitine and lipoic acid to old rats significantly improves metabolic function while decreasing oxidative stress. *Proc Natl Acad Sci,*

2002; 99:1870-1875.

30. Ames BN, et al. Mitochondrial decay in aging. *Biochim Biophys Acta,* 1995; 1271(1):165-170.

31. Tory MH, et al. Mitochondrial decay in aging: reversal through supplementation of acetyl-l-carnitine and n-tert-butyl-⊠-phenyl-nitrone. *Ann N Y Acad Sci,* 1998; 854:214-223.

32. Bruno V, et al. Protective action of idebenone against excitotoxic degeneration in cultured cortical neurons. *Neurosci Lett,* 1994; 178:193-196.

33. Napolitano A, et al. Long-term treatment with idebenone and riboflavin in a patient with MELAS. *Neurol Sci,* 2002; 21: S981-982.

34. Lerman-Sagie T, et al. Dramatic improvement in mitochondrial cardiomyopathy following treatment with idebenone. *J Inherit Metab Dis,* 2001; 24:28-34.

35. Yamada K, et al. Protective effect of idebenone and alpha-tocopherol on beta-amyloid-(1-42)-induced learning and memory deficits in ratsLimplication of oxidative stress in beta-amyloid-induced neurotoxicity in vivo. *Eur J Neurosci,* 1999; 11:83-90.

36. Gutzman H, et al. Safety and efficacy of idebenone versus tacrine in patients with Alzheimer's disease: results of a randomized, double-blind, parallel-group multicenter study. *Pharmacopsychiatry,* 2002; 35:12-18.

37. Ebadi M, et al. Neuroptotective actions of selegiline. J Neurosci Res, 2002; 67:285-289.

38. Lee CS, et al. Effect of R-(-)-deprenyl and harmaline on dopamine-and peroxyrite-induced membrane permeability transition in brain mitochondria. *Neurochem Res,* 2002; 27:215-224.

39. Pratico D, et al. Oxidative injury in diseases of the central nervous system: focus on Alzheimer's disease. *Am J Med,* 2000; 109:577-585.

40. Knoll J. Deprenyl meditation. A strategy to modulate the age related decline of

striatal dopaminergic system. *J Am Geriat Soc,* 1992; 40:839-847.

41. Schatzberg AF, et al. *Manual of Clinical Pharmacology,* 2nd Edition. Washington, DC, American Psychiatric Press, 1990.

42. Babb SM, et al. Chronic citicoline increases phosphodiesters in the brains of healthy older subjects: an in vivo phosphorus magniteic resonance spectroscopy study. *Psychopharmacology,* 2002; 161:248-254.

43. Amenta F, et al. Treatment of cognitive dysfunction associated with Alzheimer's disease with cholinergic precursors. Ineffective treatments or inappropriate approaches? *Mech Ageing* 2001; 122:2025-2040.

44. Lopez G, et al. Effects of orally administered cytidine5-diphosphate choline on brain phosolipid content. *J Nutr Biochem,* 1992; 3:313-315.

45. Adibhatla RM, et al. Citicoline: neuroprotective mechanisms in cerebral ischemia. *J Neurochem,* 2002; 80:12-23.

46. Grieb P, et al. CNP-choline, but not cytidine, protects hippocampal CA1 neurones in the gerbil following transient forebrain ischaemia. *Folia Neurophathol,* 2001; 39:141-145.

47. Clark WM, et al. A phase III randomized efficacy trial of 2000 mg citicoline in acute ischemic stroke patients. *Neurology,* 2001; 57:1595-1602.

Chapter 6: Nitric Oxide

1. Calabrese V, et al. NO synthase and NO-dependent signal pathways in brain aging and neurodegenerative disorders: the role of oxidant/antioxidant balance. *Neurochem Res,* 2000; 25:1315-1341.

2. Bashkatova VG, Rayevsky KS. Nitric oxide in mechanisms of brain damage induced by neurotoxic effect of glutamate. *Biochemistry,* 1998; 63:866-873.

3. Iadecola C, Alexander M. Cerebral ischemia and inflammation. Curr Opin Neurol, 2001; 14:89-94.

4. De Cristobal J, et al. Aspirin inhibits stress-induced increase in plasma glutamate, brain oxidative damage and ATP fall in rats. *Neuroreport*, 2002; 13:217-221.

5. Calderon-Garciduenas L, et al. Air pollution and brain damage. Toxicol Pathol, 2002; 30:373-389.

6. Calderon-Garcinuenas, et al. Brain inflammation and Alzheimer's-like pathology in individuals exposed to severe air pollution. *Toxicol Pathol*, 2004; 32: 650-658.

7. Beckman JS. The double role of nitric oxide in brain function and superoxide mediated injury. J *Dev Physiol*, 1991; 15:53-59.

8. Chan PH, et al. SOD-1 transgenic mice as a model for studies of neuroprotection in stroke and brain trauma. *Ann N Y Acad Sci*, 1994; 738:97-103.

9. Imam SZ, et al. Prevention of dopaminergic neurotoxicity by targeting nitric oxide and peroxynitrite: implications for the prevention of methamphetamine-induced neurotoxic damage. *Ann N Y Acad Sci*, 2000; 914:157-171.

10. Sugaya K. Glial activation and brain aging. *Nippon Yakurigaku Zasshi*, 2001; 118:251-257.

11. Goodwin H, et al. Microglial release of nitric oxide by the synergistic action of beta amyloid and INF-gamma. *Brain Res*, 1995; 692:207-214.

12. Tarkowski E, et al. Intrathecal release of nitric oxide in Alzheimer's disease and vascular dementia. *Dement Geriatr Cogn Disord*, 2000; 11:322-326.

13. Heales SJ, et al. Nitric oxide, mitochondria and neurological disease. *Biochim Biophys Acta*, 1999; 1410:215-228.

14. Bagastra G, et al. Activation of the inducible form of nitric oxide synthase in the brains of patients with multiple sclerosis. *Proc Nat Acad Sci*, USA, 1995; 92:12041-12045.

15. Wu DC, et al. Blockade of microglial activation is neuroprotective in the l-methyl-4-phenyl-1,2,3,6-tetrahydopyridine mouse model of Parkinson disease. *J Neurosci*, 2002; 22:1763-1771.

16. Beal MF. Mitochondria, NO and neurodegeneration. *Biochem Soc Symp*, 1999; 66:43-54.

17. Tarkowski E, et al. Intrathecal release of nitric oxide and its relation to final brain damage in patients with stroke. *Cerebrovasc Dis*, 2000; 10:200-206.

18. Raevskii KS, et al. The role of nitric oxide in brain glutaminergic pathology. *Vestn Ross Akad Med Nauk*, 2000; (4):11-15.

19. Hantraye P, et al. Inhibition of neuronal nitric oxide synthase prevents MPTP-induced Parkinsonism in baboons. *Nat Med*, 1996; 2:1017-1021.

20. Sheu F, et al. Suppression effect of soy isoflavones on nitric oxide production in RAW 264.7 macrophages. *J Agric Food Chem*, 2001; 49:1767-1772.

21. Trieu VN, Uckun FM. Genistein is neuroprotective in murine models of familial amytrophic lateral sclerosis and stroke. *Biochem Biophys Res Commun*, 1999; 258:685-688.

22. Kim H, et al. Attenuation of neurodegeneration-relevant modifications of brain proteins by dietary soy. *Biofactors*, 2000; 12:243-250.

23. Schwartz IF, et al. Garlic attenuates nitric oxide production in rat cardiac myocytes through inhibition of inducible nitric oxide synthase and the arginine transporter CAT-2 (cationic amino acid transporter-2). *Clin Sci*, 2002; 102:487-493.

24. Sun BL, et al. Effects of Gingko biloba extract on somatosensory evoked potential, nitric oxide levels in serum and brain tissue in rats with cerebral vasospasm after subarachnoid hemorrhage. *Clin Hemorheol Microcirc*, 2000; 23:139-144.

25. Le Bars PH, et al. A placebo-controlled double-blind trial of an extract of gingko biloba for dementia. *JAMA*, 1997; 278:1327-1332.

26. Sheu SY, et al. Inhibition of xanthine oxidase by purpurogallin and silymarin group. *Anti-cancer Res*, 1998; 18:263-267.

27. Cross AH, et al. Aminoquanidine, an inhibitor of inducible nitric oxide synthase ameliorates experimental encephalopathies in SIL Mice. *Clin Invest*, 1994;

93:2684-2690.

28. Perlmutter D. Functional therapies in neurodegenerative disease. *J Appl Nutr*, 1999; 51:3-13.

29. Saito K, Yoshioka H. Protective effect of spin trap agent, N-tert-butyl-alpha-phenylnitrone on hyperoxia-induced oxidative stress and its potential as a nitric oxide donor. Free Rad Res, 2002; 36:143-149.

30. Floyd RA. Antioxidants, oxidative stress, and degenerative neurological disorders. Proc Soc E*xp Biol Med*, 1999; 222:236-245.

Chapter 7: The Brain in Flames

1. Bain BE, Chirinas–Rojas Ch. COX-2 inhibitors: Current perceptions and future opportunities. *Physician Forum*, 2002; 1:1-121. www.dresources.com

2. MacLean P. *The Triune Brain In Evolution*. New York: Plenum Press, 1990.

3. De Cristobal J, et al. Aspirin inhibits stress-induced increase in plasma glutamate, brain oxidative damage and ATP fall in rats. *Neuroreport*, 2002; 13:217-221.

4. Calderon-Garciduenas L, et al. Air pollution and brain damage. Toxicol Pathol, 2002; 30:373-389.

5. *US National Vital Statistics Report*, 2002; 50:7-10.

6. Stewart WF, et al. Risk of Alzheimer's disease and duration of NSAID use. *Neurology*, 1997; 48:626-632.

7. Veld BA, et al. Now-steroidal anit-inflammatory drugs and the risk of Alzheimer's disease. *New Engl J Med*, 2001; 345:1515-1521.

8. Vane JR, Botting RM. Mechanism of action of nonsteroidal anti-inflammatory drugs. *Am J Med*, 1998; 104:2S-8S.

9. Brune K. Next generation of everyday analgesics. *Am J Ther*, 2002; 9:215-223.

10. Sooriakumaran P. COX-2 inhibitors and the heart: are all coxibs the same? *Postgrad Medi J*, 2006; 62:242-245.

11. Topol, E. "Arthritis Medications and Cardiovascular Events – "House of Coxibs." *JAMA*, 2005; 293:366-369.

12. Surh YJ, et al. Molecular mechanisms underlying chemopreventive activities of anti inflammatory phytochemicals: down regulation of COX-2 and INOS through suppression of NF-kappa B activation. *Mutat Res,* 2001; 480:243-268.

13. Surh YJ. Anti-tumor promoting potential of selected spice ingredients and anti inflammatory activities: a short review. *Food Chem Toxicol,* 2002; 40:1091-1097.

14. Reddy BS, Rao CV. Novel approaches for colon cancer prevention by cyclooxygenase-2 inhibitors. *J Environ Pathol Toxicol Oncol,* 2002; 21:155-164.

15. Goel A, et al. Specific inhibition of cyclooxygenase-2 (COX-2) expression by dietary curcumin in HT29 human colon cancer cells. *Cancer Lett,* 2001; 172:111-118.

16. Lee SK, et al. Supressive effect of natural sesquiterpenoids on inducible cyclooxegenase and nitric oxide synthase activity in mouse macrophage cells. *J Environ Pathol Toxicol Oncol,* 2002; 21:141-148.

17. Khan A, et al. Cinnamon improves glucose and lipids of people with type 2 diabetes. *Diabetes Care,* 2003; 26:3215-3218.

18. Anderson R, et al. Insulin and cinnamon polyphenols increase the amount of insulin receptor beta, glucose transporter 4, anti-inflammatory protein tristetraprolin in mouse 3T3-L1 adipocytes. Paper presented at the *Experimental Biology Conference,* 2006; San Francisco:April 1-5.

19. Lampke S, et al. Activation of insulin-like activity of proanthocyanidins from cinnamon. Paper presented a the *Experimental Biology Conference,* 2006; San Francisco:April 1-5.

20. Fuhrman B, et al. Ginger extract consumption reduces plasma cholesterol, inhibits LDL oxidation, an attenuates development of atherosclerosis in atherosclerotic, apolipoprotein E-deficient mice. *J Nutr,* 2000 ; 130(5):1124-1131.

21. Grzanna R, et al.   Ginger-an herbal medicinal product with broad anti-inflammatory actions. *J Med Food*, 2005; 8(2):125-132.

22. Lee M, et al.   Eugenol inhibits calcium currents in dental afferent neurons. *Dent Res*, 2005; 84(9):848-851.

23. Khan A, et al.   Cloves improve glucose cholesterol and triglycerides of people with Type 2 diabetes paper presented at the *Experimental Biology Conference San Francisco*; 2006: April 1-5.

24. Szolcsanyi J.   Forty years in spsaicin research for sensory pharmacology and physiology. *Neuropeptides*, 2004; 38(6):377-384.

25. Szolcsanyi J, et al.   Systemic anti-inflammatory effect induced by counter-irritation throu somatosatin from nocicptors. *British J Pharmacology*, 1998; 125:916-922.

26. Kelly VE, et al.   A fish oil diet rich in eicosapentaenoic acid reduces cyclooxygenase metabolites and suppresses lupus in MRL-lpr mice. *J Immunol*, 1985; 134:1914-1919.

27. Tomobe Y, et al.   Dietary Docosahexaenoic acid suppresses inflammation and immunoresponses in contact hypersensitivity reaction in mice.   *Lipids*, 2000; 35:61-69.

Chapter 8: Parkinson's Puzzle

1.   Parkinson J. An essay on the shaking palsy. 1817. Reproduced in *J. Neuropsychiatry Clin Neurosci*, 2002; 14(2):223-236.

2.   Parkinson Society Canada.   www.parkinson.ca/research/research.html.   Accessed 20 August 2006.

3.   Veldman BA, et al.   Genetic and environmental risk factors in Parkinson's disease. *Clin Neurol Neurosurg*, 1998; 100(1):15-26.

4.   Semchuk RM, et al.   Parkinson's disease and exposure to agricultural work and pesticide chemicals. Neurology, 1992; 42:1328-1335.

5. Czlonkowska A, Kurkowska-Jastrzebska I. Treatment of neurodegenerative diseases: new perspectives. *Neurol Neurochir Pol,* 2001; 35(4 Suppl):147-156.

6. Wu DC, et al. Blockade of microglial activation is neuroprotective in the l-methyl-4-phenyl-1,2,3,6-tetrahydropyridine mouse model of Parkinson disease. *J Neurosci,* 2002; 22(5):1763-1771.

7. Calabrese V, et al. Mitochondrial involvement in brain function and dysfunction: relevance to aging, neurodegenerative disorders and longevity. *Neurochem Res,* 2001; 26(6):739-764.

8. The Michael J Fox Foundation. www.michaeljfox.org. Accessed 20 August 2006.

9. Forno LS. Neuropathology of Parkinson's disease. *J Neuropathol Exp Neurol,* 1996; 55:259-272.

10. Lai BCL, et al. The prevalence of Parkinsons's disease in British Columbia, Canada, estimated by using drug tracer methodology. *Parkinsonism and Related Disorders,* 2003; 9:233-241.

11. Natural Institute of Neurological Disorders. What is dementia with Lewy bodies? www.ninds.nih.gov/disorders. Accessed 20 August 2006.

12. Baldi I, et al. Neuropsychologic effects of long-term exposure to pesticides: results from the French Phytoner study. *Environ Health Perspect,* 2001; 109:839-844.

13. Thiruchelvam M, et al. Developmental exposure to the pesticides paraquat and maneb and the Parkinson's disease phenotype. *Neurotoxicology,* 2002; 23:621-633.

14. Barlow BK, et al. Neurotoxicology, 2005; 26(1):63-75.

15. Ascharis A, et al. Pesticides exposure associated with Parkinson's disease. www.sciencedaily.com. Accessed 21 August 2006.

16. Lee DW, Opanashuk LA. Polychlorinated biphenyl mixture aroclor 1254-induced oxidative stress plays a role in dopaminergic cell injury. *Neurotoxicology,* 2004;

25(6):925-939.

17. Lee DW, et al. Heme-oxygenase-1 promotes polychlorinated biphenyl mixture arochlor 1254-induced oxidative stress and dopaminergic cell injury. *Toxicol Sci*, 2006; 90(1):159-167.

18. Ross GW et al. Association of coffee and caffeine intake with the risk of Parkinson's. *JAMA*, 2000; 283:2674-2679.

19. Ascherio A, et al. Prospective study of caffeine consumption and risk of Parkinson's disease in men and women.

Chapter 9: Alzheimer's Alert

1. Alzheimer A. *JAMA*, 1969; 208:1017-1018.

2. Alzheimer A. Uber einen eigenartigen schweren Krankheitrsprozess der Hirnrinde Zontralblatt fur Nervenkrankheiten. 1906; 25:1134.

3. Naslund J, et al. Correlation between elevated levels of amyloid beta-peptide in the brain and cognitive decline. *JAMA*, 2000; 283:1571-1576.

4. Green MS, et al. The Oregon Brain Aging Study. *Neurology*, 2000; 54:105-113.

5. American Alzheimer's Association. www.alz.org. Accessed 20 August 2006.

6. Canadian Alzheimer's Society. www.alzheimer.ca. Accessed 20 August 2006.

7. US National Institute on Aging. www.nia.nih.gov/Alzheimers. Accessed 20 August 2006.

8. *US National Vital Statistics Report*, 2002, 50, 7-10.

9. Hebert, LE, et al. Alzheimer disease in the US population: Prevalence estimates using the 2000 census. *Arch Neurol*, 2003; 60:1119-1122.

10. US National Institutes of Health. *Progress Report on Alzheimer's Disease*, 2000. www.alzheimers.org/pub/prog. Accessed 6 September 2006.

11. Peterson RC, et al. Memory and MRI-based hippocampul volume in aging and AD. *Neurology*, 2000; 54:581-587.

12. Killiany RJ, et al. Use of structural magnetic resonance imagery to predict who will get Alzheimer's disease. *Ann Neurol*, 2000; 47:430-439.

13. Fox NC, et al. Using serial registered brain magnetic resonance imaging to measure disease progression in Alzheimer's disease. *Arch Neurol*, 2000; 57:339-344.

14. Pronczuk J, et al. Global perspectives in breast milk contamination: infections and toxic hazards. *Environ Health Perspect*, 2002; 110:A349-351.

15. Landrigan PJ, et al. Chemical contaminants in breast milk and their impacts on children's health: an overview. *Environ Health Perspect*, 2002; 110(6):A313-5.

16. Uboga NV, Price JI. Formation of diffuse and fibrillar tangles in aging and early Alzheimer's disease. *Neurobiology of Aging*, 2000; 21:1-10.

17. Ishihara T, et al. Age-dependent emergence and progression of tauopathy in mice expressing the shortest human tau isoform. *Neuron*, 1999; 24:751-762.

18. Lewis J, et al. Neurofibrillary tangles, amyotrophy and progressive motor disturbance in mice expressing mutant (P3OIL) tau protein. *Nature Genetics*, 2000; 25:402-405.

19. Trojanowski, JQ. Neuropathological verisimilitude in animal models of Alzheimer's disease. *Am J Pathol*, 2002; 160:409-411.

20. Troy CM, et al. Caspase-2 mediates neuronal cell death induced by beta-amyloid. *J Neurosci*, 2000; 20:1386-1392.

21. Harman D. Alzheimer's disease: role of aging in pathogenesis. *Ann N Y Acad* Sci, 2002; 959:384-395.

22. 22.Hagen TM, et al. (R) alpha lipoic acid – supplemented old rats have improved mitochondrial function, decreased oxidative damage and increased metabolic rate. *FASEB*, 1999; 13:411-418.

23. Meier-Ruge W, et al. Changes in brain glucose metabolism as a key to the pathogenesis of Alzheimer's disease. *Gerontology*, 1994; 246-252.

Chapter 10: The Brain Program

1. Bankston J. *Joseph Lister and the Story of Antiseptics.* London: Mitchell Lane, 2004.

2. Juliano LM, Griffiths, RR. A critical review of caffeine withdrawal: empirical validation of symptoms and signs, incidence severity, and associated features. *Psychopharmacology* 2004; 176(1):1-29.

3. Colgan M. *The New Nutrition.* Vancouver: Apple Publishing, 1996.

4. Colgan M. *Hormonal Health.* Vancouver: Apple Publishing, 1996.

5. Colgan M. *The New Power Program.* Vancouver: Apple Publishing, 2001.

6. Landrigan PJ, et al. Health and Environmental Consequences of the World Trade Center Disaster. *Environmental Health Perspectives*, 2004; 112:731-739. www.mindfully.org/Air/2004/WTC-Health-Consequences1may04.htm; accessed 11 September 2006.

7. *Science Daily.* www.sciencedaily.com. Accessed 11 September 2006.

8. *Law Enforcement News.* www.officer.com. Accessed 11 September 2006.

9. Eto K. Minamata disease. *Neuropathology*, 2000; 20(s1):14-19.

10. Eto K. Pathology of Minamata disease. *Toxicol Pathol*, 1997; 25(6):614-623.

Chapter 11: A Quiet Mind

1. Colgan M. *Nutrition for Champions.* Vancouver: Science Books, 2007.

2. Eaton SB. An evolutionary perspective enhances understanding of humqan nutritional requirements. *J Nutr*, 1996. 126 1732-1140.

3. National Center for Health Statistics. www.cdc.gov.nchs, Accessed 20 September 2006.

4. Skaer TL, et al. Trends in the use of antidepressant pharmacotherapy and diagnosis of depression in the US. *CNS Drugs*, 2000; 14: 473-481.

5. Friedman H (Ed) *Psychoneuroimmunology, Stress and Infectious Disease,* Boca Raton, FL:CRC Press, 1996.

6. Claxton G. *The Heart of Buddhism,* Thorsons, 1992.

7. Suzuki DT. *Zen and Japanese Culture,* Princeton University Press, 1993.

8. Hassnain FM. *A Search For The Historical Jesus.* London: Gateway Books, 1994.

9. Prophet EC. *The Lost Years of Jesus.* Livingston MT: Summit University Press, 1987.

10. Notovitch N. *The Unknown Life of Jesus Christ.* Paris: Olendorf, 1894.

11. Deardorff JW. *A new ecumenism based on reexamination of the lost years evidence..* Portland: Oregon State University, September 2003.

Index

A

Dr. Michael Colgan

Michael Colgan, PhD, CCN, is an internationally renowned research scientist. He is acknowledged as one of the world's most popular scientific experts in nutrition, exercise and the inhibition of aging.

From 1971 to 1982, Dr. Colgan was a senior member of the Science Faculty of the University of Auckland, where he taught in Human Sciences and conducted research on aging and physical performance. Startling results of his early research convinced him to write his first book for the public, Your Personal Vitamin Profile, during his tenure as a visiting scholar at Rockefeller University in New York. This revolutionary book rapidly became a definitive guide for accurate, scientifically researched nutritional information.

From 1979 to 1998, Dr. Colgan was the Director and President of the Colgan Institute; now he serves as Chairman of the Board. The Colgan Institute has branches in the United States, Canada and Australasia. The Colgan Institute is a consulting, educational and research facility founded in 1979, primarily concerned with the effects of nutrition and exercise on athletic performance, aging and the prevention of degenerative disease.

Dr. Colgan has served as a consultant to the US National Institute on Aging and to the New Zealand and Canadian Governments, as well as many corporations. His professional memberships include the American Academy of Anti-Aging Medicine, the American College of Sports Medicine, the New York Academy of Sciences, the British Society for Nutritional Medicine, and the International and American Associations of Clinical Nutritionists (IAACN). In 2002 Dr. Colgan was inducted into the Canadian Sports Nutrition Hall of Fame.

With a distinguished reputation for his expertise in sports nutrition, Dr. Colgan has advised hundreds of athletes of all abilities and ages throughout the world. These include track and field Olympians Donovan Bailey, Quincy Watts, Leroy Burrell, Steve Scott, Michelle Burrell, Meredith Rainey Valmon and Regina Jacobs; three-time world boxing champion Bobby Czyz; rowers Francis Reininger and Adrian Cassidy; powerlifter Rick Roberts; two-time world triathlon champion Julie Moss and world-class triathlete Brandyn Gray; shooting champion T'ai Erasmus; Australian heavyweight boxing champion Chris Sharpe; motorcross champion Danny Smith; and bodybuilding champions Lee Labrada, Lee Haney and Lenda Murray.

For more information on Dr. Colgan and the Colgan Institute, as well as information on Colgan Institute products, programs, and upcoming events, visit www.colganinstitute.com.

Cartoons

The cartoons in this book and others in each series are available for purchase as follows:

Caveman and Humor Series:
High resolution digital image on disc for one time use in newsletters and magazines, Black and White $29.95, Full Color $39.95 each.

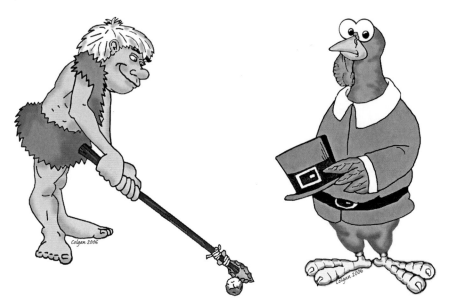

Limited Edition Prints:
Matt limited edition prints from any series, full color, 8" x 10", signed by the artist and mounted $89.95 each.

For 11" x17" prints, please contact The Colgan Institute for details

Political and Celebrity Series:

High resolution digital image on disc for one time use in newsletters and magazines, Black and White $49.95, Full Color $69.95 each.

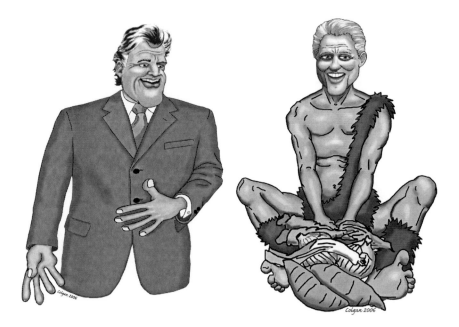

Authors or Publishers wishing to publish cartoons from any series in books please phone or email for contract.

Colgan Institute Canada Ltd

988 North End Rd, Salt Spring Island
BC, Canada, V8K 1L7
Ph: 250 537 2069 email: admin@colganinstitute.com
Fax: 250 537 5824 website: www.colganinstitute.com

All prices in Canadian dollars and subject to all applicable taxes. The Colgan Institute reserves the right to change prices and availability without notice.